Professor Robert Bor is a director of Dynamic Change Consultants, and Lead Clinical Psychologist in Medical Specialities at the Royal Free Hospital, London. A Chartered Clinical, Counselling and Health Psychologist registered with the UK Health and Care Professions Council, he is also a Fellow of the British Psychological Society and Member of the American Psychological Association, and has over 29 years' experience consulting in clinical and organizational settings in the UK and abroad. He is a UKCP registered Family and Couples Therapist, having specialized in systemic therapy at the Tavistock Clinic, London. Rob also practises cognitive behavioural therapy and is an advocate of time-limited and solution-focused therapeutic approaches. He works with children, adolescents, adults, couples, families and teams within organizations, and is Consulting Psychologist to the Leaders in Oncology Care and to the London Clinic (both in Harley Street). He also provides psychological consultations and executive coaching to organizations such as PwC and UBS, among others, in London and abroad. He is consulting psychologist to St Paul's School, the Royal Ballet School and JFS in London. Rob is an Accredited Aviation Psychologist and also Honorary Civilian Psychologist to the Royal Air Force. He holds the Freedom of the City of London and is a Churchill Fellow.

Dr Carina Eriksen is a Chartered and UK Health and Care Professions Council registered Counselling Psychologist with an extensive London-based private practice for young people, adults, couples and families. She is a consultant with Dynamic Change Consultants and an accredited member of the British Association for Behavioural and Cognitive Psychotherapies, having specialized at the Institute of Psychiatry. Carina has managed a team of psychologists, CBT therapists and psychotherapists in the NHS for several years and was previously an external supervisor at The Priory. She has extensive experience consulting in clinical and organizational settings in the UK and Europe. Carina is a consultant at Colet Court, the preparatory school for St Paul's School for Boys, and works closely with several British and international schools in London. She is actively involved in research, with a specific interest in the topic of work stress and work–life balance, anxiety, panic, fear of flying, and the psychological effects of living with cancer. Carina and her colleagues are often invited to present these topics at conferences in the UK and abroad. ·

Dr Sara Chaudry is a Chartered Counselling Psychologist registered with the UK Health and Care Professions Council and the British Psychological Society. Sara has a broad range of clinical experience derived from working in various contexts including the NHS, private practice, schools and charitable organizations. She has gained a wealth of experience from working with diverse client groups that include adults, couples, children, adolescents and families. Sara also provides therapy for individuals employed in various organizations based in ⸻ ⸻don. Her work draws from various influential psychological mode⸻ and influenced by cognitive behavioural therapy. ⸻ visiting lecturer at City University London.

Overcoming Common Problems Series

Selected titles

A full list of titles is available from Sheldon Press,
36 Causton Street, London SW1P 4ST and on our website at
www.sheldonpress.co.uk

Overcoming Common Problems Series

Overcoming Common Problems Series

Living with Physical Disability and Amputation
Dr Keren Fisher

Living with Schizophrenia
Dr Neel Burton and Dr Phil Davison

Living with a Stoma
Professor Craig A. White

Living with Tinnitus and Hyperacusis
Dr Laurence McKenna, Dr David Baguley
and Dr Don McFerran

Losing a Parent
Fiona Marshall

**Making Sense of Trauma: How to tell
your story**
Dr Nigel C. Hunt and Dr Sue McHale

Menopause in Perspective
Philippa Pigache

Motor Neurone Disease: A family affair
Dr David Oliver

The Multiple Sclerosis Diet Book
Tessa Buckley

Natural Treatments for Arthritis
Christine Craggs-Hinton

Overcome Your Fear of Flying
Professor Robert Bor, Dr Carina Eriksen
and Margaret Oakes

Overcoming Agoraphobia
Melissa Murphy

Overcoming Anorexia
Professor J. Hubert Lacey, Christine
Craggs-Hinton and Kate Robinson

Overcoming Emotional Abuse
Susan Elliot-Wright

Overcoming Fear: With mindfulness
Deborah Ward

**Overcoming Gambling: A guide for problem
and compulsive gamblers**
Philip Mawer

Overcoming Hurt
Dr Windy Dryden

Overcoming Jealousy
Dr Windy Dryden

Overcoming Loneliness
Alice Muir

**Overcoming Panic and Related Anxiety
Disorders**
Margaret Hawkins

Overcoming Procrastination
Dr Windy Dryden

Overcoming Shyness and Social Anxiety
Dr Ruth Searle

**The Pain Management Handbook:
Your personal guide**
Neville Shone

The Panic Workbook
Dr Carina Eriksen, Professor Robert Bor
and Margaret Oakes

**Physical Intelligence: How to take charge
of your weight**
Dr Tom Smith

Reducing Your Risk of Dementia
Dr Tom Smith

**Self-discipline: How to get it
and how to keep it**
Dr Windy Dryden

The Self-Esteem Journal
Alison Waines

Sinusitis: Steps to healing
Dr Paul Carson

Stammering: Advice for all ages
Renée Byrne and Louise Wright

Stress-related Illness
Dr Tim Cantopher

Ten Steps to Positive Living
Dr Windy Dryden

**Therapy for Beginners: How to get the best
out of counselling**
Professor Robert Bor, Sheila Gill and Anne Stokes

Think Your Way to Happiness
Dr Windy Dryden and Jack Gordon

**Tranquillizers and Antidepressants:
When to take them, how to stop**
Professor Malcolm Lader

**Transforming Eight Deadly Emotions
into Healthy Ones**
Dr Windy Dryden

The Traveller's Good Health Guide
Dr Ted Lankester

Treating Arthritis Diet Book
Margaret Hills

Treating Arthritis: The drug-free way
Margaret Hills and Christine Horner

Treating Arthritis: More ways to a drug-free life
Margaret Hills

Treating Arthritis: The supplements guide
Julia Davies

Understanding Obsessions and Compulsions
Dr Frank Tallis

Understanding Traumatic Stress
Dr Nigel Hunt and Dr Sue McHale

The User's Guide to the Male Body
Jim Pollard

When Someone You Love Has Dementia
Susan Elliot-Wright

**When Someone You Love Has Depression:
A handbook for family and friends**
Barbara Baker

Overcoming Common Problems

Overcoming Stress

PROFESSOR ROBERT BOR,
DR CARINA ERIKSEN
AND DR SARA CHAUDRY

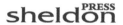

First published in Great Britain in 2014

Sheldon Press
36 Causton Street
London SW1P 4ST
www.sheldonpress.co.uk

The authors and publisher have made every effort to ensure that the external
website and email addresses included in this book are correct and up to date at the
time of going to press. The authors and publisher are not responsible for the content,
quality or continuing accessibility of the sites.

British Library Cataloguing-in-Publication Data
A catalogue record for this book is available from the British Library

ISBN 978-1-84709-266-3
eBook ISBN 978-1-84709-267-0

Typeset by Caroline Waldron, Wirral, Cheshire
First printed in Great Britain by Ashford Colour Press
Subsequently digitally reprinted in Great Britain

eBook by Fakenham Prepress Solutions, Fakenham, Norfolk NR21 8NN

Produced on paper from sustainable forests

Contents

1

Introduction

If you are reading this book you are probably seeking to understand the nature of stress and how best to overcome it. You may have little interest in the benefits or advantages of stress in your life – you may simply feel that your stress has exceeded the point where you can continue to cope. Before we go on to deal with overcoming stress, however, we would very briefly like to highlight some of the *positive* aspects of stress to help you understand that, despite what we are led to believe, not all stress is inherently bad.

Stress can boost your brainpower, galvanize you, and help to keep you alert and engaged in what is going on around you. It can have secondary benefits as well, helping to enhance your self-esteem, your confidence and your personal achievements. It can even help to bring out the best in you when dating or choosing a life partner by keeping you focused on making a good impression and presenting yourself as positively as you can.

This book, however, will focus not on the advantages and benefits of stress (we can probably assume that these are unlikely to trouble most readers!) but rather on the negative effects which stress can have on us.

When we experience stress we can be aware of unpleasant physical sensations and thought patterns which hold us back and cause us to worry. Of course, much depends on how we experience the feelings caused by stress. Stress is however extremely common and negatively affects everyone at one time or another.

For a certain proportion of people – children as well as adults – stress can be a recurrent feature in their life, even a daily ordeal. There may be times when our levels of stress are such that we feel overburdened or incapacitated, whether in our personal lives, at work, or in relation to hobbies, achievements or social interaction. In some circumstances we may experience several different sources of stress at the same time, and this cumulative burden can make it difficult for us to see even how to begin to overcome stress.

All of this can make us feel vulnerable and anxious about ourselves and, in turn, can affect our body's functioning. An accumulation of negatively experienced stress can also affect our mood, our sleep and our general well-being. This, of course, can all lead us to experience even greater stress.

Our experience with people who suffer from stress shows that some have a good understanding of how stress affects them – but do not necessarily have the particular skills and techniques they need in order to overcome their stress. One reason for this may be that each of us has a different threshold for stress and can be affected differently by it. A variety of situations give rise to stress, and for some people a single situation may be a major challenge while for others stress only occurs when there is a cumulative effect, one stressful situation after another.

Our aim in this book is therefore to help you to understand the nature and effects of negatively experienced stress, physical as well as mental, and to gain insight into how this type of stress has different effects on different people. We will show you how some of our clients have described their own experiences with stress and its often far-reaching impact on their lives. These case studies will help you to reflect on your own experience of stress and lead you towards solutions. We will also help you to understand how stress builds up, and the importance of using countermeasures in order to relieve this build-up and prevent it becoming overwhelming or incapacitating. We outline the way in which stress becomes an issue in the first place, and help you to identify and detect early signs so that you are in a position to prevent the escalation of stress.

We also describe methods by which you can cope with and finally overcome stress. We will show you how to select and practise the techniques most likely to help you successfully overcome stress in your life.

The problem of stress

Stress has a serious impact on the physical and psychological well-being of a substantial proportion of the adult population. A recent (2012) Mental Health Foundation survey found that 47 per cent of people feel stressed every day or every few days, and 59 per cent feel that their lives are more stressful than they were five years ago.

It is far more complicated, and arguably less precise, to measure stress than to measure, say, body temperature or blood pressure. The reason for this is that with stress, subjectivity – a personal tolerance effect – enters the equation. All of us know people who thrive on high levels of stress and appear to do well when under pressure. Indeed, they may actually underperform when they are not functioning under stress. For others, the complete opposite may apply; for such people, situations which most people tolerate with relative ease, such as leaving home to go shopping, may present overwhelming levels of stress.

Whatever levels of stress you may be experiencing, it is unhelpful – and arguably wrong – for others to judge whether the stress you are suffering is acceptable or unacceptable, good or bad, and whether your stress is intense or mild. Only you and/or a professional counsellor can make this decision.

Stress is generally considered unwelcome, even if we do thrive on it in the short term. It is easy to see that too much stress can have a negative impact on our physical health and on our work and personal lives. Prolonged episodes of stress can lead to inflammation in parts of the body and susceptibility to infection. Prolonged stress also increases our risk of experiencing more serious and debilitating psychological conditions, such as chronic anxiety, panic attacks and depression – and serious physical health problems such as coronary heart disease, high blood pressure, gastric conditions including irritable bowel syndrome, and even diabetes.

For the most part, however – you will probably be very glad to know – stress is preventable, manageable and treatable. Of course there are situations, whether personal or work-related, where part of the reason we are experiencing stress is because we feel powerless to change the circumstances in which we find ourselves. For example, if we fear losing a job, in the current economic climate we are more likely to be very sensitive and responsive to the hints and expectations of a boss to work longer hours or take on extra tasks with no extra benefits. Understanding the conditions in which we find ourselves, even though we are unable to change some or all of the aspects of a situation, can help us to cope better with the stress the situation is causing for us. There are very likely to be things we can do in order to alleviate some of the stress in our working day.

In our experience, and from the research which has been published on the subject of coping with stress, there is consensus that everyone should be able to do something to reduce stress in their lives provided they have properly understood its source and cause, and what is maintaining it, using modern psychological methods.

What is different about this book?

There have been numerous books published on coping with stress – so why have we written another one? There are several reasons, and a number of ways in which you might find this book different.

First, the book brings together the latest proven methods for overcoming stress, methods which have been tried and tested with real patients in a professional clinical setting. These are methods our patients have used successfully to overcome their stress. We also provide you with techniques which are unique and specific to you, and which will help you to find your particular key to unlocking your understanding of your stress and so help you to prevent or overcome it.

Second, it is written by a highly experienced and uniquely qualified team of psychologists who have extensive experience in working with people who suffer from stress, whether in the workplace or in their personal lives. All three of us work with people employed in the financial and legal sectors of the City of London, and with people who have severe and even life-threatening health problems, as well as with children, families and adults who experience stress in their day-to-day lives. Not only do we understand how stress affects people in all areas of their lives, meaning that we are able to pool our knowledge and resources, but each of us is qualified as a general psychologist – together, we have more than fifty years' professional experience – and therefore we have assessed and treated a wide range of other psychological difficulties. We are all aware of and sensitive to the impact of stress in people's everyday lives, as well as its psychological effects. We have published our research findings in specialist medical and psychological journals as well as in books, and we are often invited to talk about stress at conferences around the world. So the tailored approach to self-help taken in this book is built on a solid foundation of clinical practice and research.

Third, reflecting our approach to the treatment of stress, the book takes a slightly different approach from other self-help books on the topic. We will not baffle you with statistics, and will certainly not convey the idea that stress is a reflection of poor self-management or an indication of personal weakness. Our starting point is that stress is ever-present and everyone experiences some measure of it. Even as professionals in the field, we ourselves are not immune to stress or its effects, and each of us has his or her own experience of stress in our personal and professional lives. So our understanding of stress is not taken solely from textbooks and research, but is a reflection of our own experience as well as that of our clients.

Fourth, we approach your stress as unique and specific, something which may differ from other people's. You will see, from the clinical examples we quote, that stress affects people in many different ways; we tailor the solutions to your unique situation. We also understand that not everyone is affected equally by stress. We are not exponents of a 'one-size-fits-all' approach to treating stress. Our experience has taught us that it is essential, in the context of psychological therapy, first of all to listen very carefully to individuals' accounts of their difficulties with stress. Of course, it is not possible to 'listen' to a personal story from the reader of a book; however, in the book we depict the diverse contexts and struggles that our clients have recounted to us, so you are very likely to find in the story of someone we have treated a situation that reflects your own.

Finally, the primary focus of this book is on the psychological skills and techniques that you can apply to overcoming stress in your life. These skills and techniques are derived from the findings of modern psychological research in cognitive behavioural therapy, systemic therapy, mindfulness-based cognitive therapy and rational-emotive therapy. The focus is on what you can *do* and how you can *think* and *feel* about different situations so as to help you on your way. You will be able to see and measure your progress each step of the way. Our approach will focus on what is happening to you now (not in your distant childhood, you may be relieved to hear!) and what you can do to bring about change.

So what's in the rest of this book?

The rest of this book contains information, techniques to practise, and advice. You will find guidance on how to select and try out the techniques most likely to work for you. The book is almost entirely practical in its focus, and is oriented towards helping you first of all to understand the source or cause of your stress from a psychological perspective. We describe in detail the different ways in which stress manifests itself. The case studies we share throughout the book illustrate the ways in which people with whom we have worked have found stress difficult and how they have overcome their negative experience of it. These examples are based on real situations and people, but we have obviously changed details which might identify them in order to preserve confidentiality.

The book goes on to highlight the wide variety of triggers which must be identified and treated in order to overcome this challenge. We emphasize throughout the importance of social context and how each of us is confronted with stressful situations but reacts in different ways. Finally we cover the information, skills and techniques you will need to begin formulating your own individual treatment and prevention strategy. By the end of the book we hope you will have gained an understanding of your own experience of stress and how it affects you, and also of how to concentrate on putting ideas into practice in order to overcome your stress.

The book is, we hope, written in a user-friendly and jargon-free style. A criticism sometimes levelled at psychologists is that, at times, we refer to concepts and terms that may not be familiar to many people. We have tried to avoid jargon and instead to focus on what is practical and usable. It is helpful to understand a bit more about the background and causes of stress if treatment is to be effective. We aim to help this process by avoiding terms and language that feels alienating or unfamiliar.

How to get the most from this book

This book is designed to help you to gain confidence and acquire the proven techniques and skills needed to overcome stress. It will engage you in reflection and encourage you to try out new skills and tasks. Since it is important to undertake an individual assessment of your stress, we will help you to understand your own way of thinking about stress and enable you to select and try out the psychological techniques that are most likely to help you to overcome it.

If you are working through the book on your own (or with a friend or relative), there are some things you can do to ensure that the time and effort you invest in the process is as rewarding as possible. A good starting point is to decide when and where you will work on your stress problem. Choose your time and place so that you can read and think comfortably and without interruption. You may find it useful to make regular short 'appointments' with yourself and put them in your diary just as you would a meeting with someone else. Or you might read the book while commuting, or during a work lunchtime. If you do choose one of these options, if your work is a source of your stress there may be some benefit in applying what you have learned immediately in that setting.

Remember that learning a new skill or technique takes practice, so half an hour a day for a week or two is likely to be more effective than a 'blitz' at the weekend. You will also find it helpful to have a notebook with you each time you have a session with the book, so you can make notes and reminders for yourself as you work through it.

At various points in each chapter you will find exercises, denoted by the 'Stop and Think' symbol:

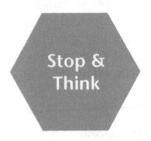

These exercises are designed to help you apply the information and techniques given in the chapter to your own situation. It can be very tempting to want to skip over these exercises as you read and tackle them later, but it is best to do them as you progress through the book. They are specifically designed to help you reflect on the accompanying material and practise the techniques we describe as you come to understand them. Use your notebook to record your reflections as well as to practise.

As stress varies widely and from person to person, no one book can cover everything that everyone needs. What we can do, however, is to outline the psychological strategies, skills and techniques which are most likely to work, and show you how to use them. Once you have been introduced to these methods, you can then try them out for yourself.

You may find that some of the ideas you come across are helpful to you in other areas of your life which present a challenge to you. We are interested not only in how people are affected by stress but, in turn, how it impacts on those around them. We find that for our clients there is sometimes a circular relationship between stress and the attitudes and beliefs of their families or work colleagues. (We will say more about the context in which stress occurs in subsequent chapters, as we believe this is important in understanding the cause, maintenance and treatment of stress.)

What if I need more help?

Sometimes in clinical settings we meet people who find that taking the first step to get psychological help for their stress was too big a challenge. Ironically, they can fear overcoming stress because they have become accustomed to it. They worry that if they are not experiencing stress then they are not performing well or taking life's challenges seriously. As unpleasant as stress can be, it can also be addictive or compulsive.

For some people stress can be deep-seated, and the effects destructive. People like this may feel that results from therapy (self-help or professional) are not coming quickly enough. If the behaviour you are targeting for change has not shifted in spite of your best efforts and having worked through this book, re-examining the nature of your difficulties rather than concluding that there must be something more serious, or even untreatable, about you is the next step. There could be several reasons why success has not come as quickly as you had hoped, and we look at these more closely in Chapter 9. You might also want to use other sources of information, or seek professional help from a therapist or counsellor, and we have provided a list of 'Useful addresses' at the end of the book that will assist you in doing so.

The ideas presented in this book are based on tried and tested methods. They come from the experience that we and many colleagues use to help treat people with stress. The book is not full of theory and textbook ideas; rather it is a practical companion to help you to understand and address your difficulties. We wish you luck in your efforts to overcome stress, and we hope that you enjoy working through the book. You have already made the first move towards understanding and overcoming your stress. This motivation will help to bring about success in return for your hard work!

2

What is stress?

Stress is probably the most common example of what is known as a psychological difficulty – something distinct from a definable psychological problem, such as clinical depression or panic disorder. We tend to say we are feeling stressed when we feel that the demands being made on us are greater than our ability to cope with them. Stress is therefore often associated with feeling under extensive or sustained pressure, and being either overwhelmed or overloaded by demands or feelings.

Stress is termed a 'difficulty' for the following reasons:

1 It is extremely common. Arguably, almost everyone experiences and reports negative stress at some stage in their life.
2 It essentially reflects a state of feelings and capacity; it can impact on behaviour but does not always do so.
3 It is a state which is relative and affects each individual differently. Some people thrive on stress, or have a high capacity for dealing with difficult situations and do not report feeling distressed in them, while others recognize stress in themselves even in the absence of any stressful situation.
4 It is hard to measure and define clearly. Unlike blood pressure or body temperature, or even depression, measurement of stress is imprecise and largely relies on the subjective and personal experience of the individual in describing it.

Stress should not, however, be treated lightly when it does occur. If stress is left untreated, it can lead to health and psychological problems which may be more extensive, more debilitating, and possibly more difficult to treat. Stress can therefore be an early warning sign that all is not entirely well and comfortable with us.

Stress directly affects our physiological state, our thoughts and our behaviour. It also has secondary effects that run the gamut from how we relate to people, our well-being and day-to-day living, our bodily patterns and functioning, to our ability to achieve our personal goals.

It is important to emphasize that stress is *not* a sign of personal weakness or an indication that we are mentally ill. Instead we need to recognize that stress affects everyone at some time; it affects both genders equally, and affects people across the full age spectrum from children to the elderly. Frequently stress is a temporary or transient state and is therefore something we will experience intermittently during our lifetime. We particularly associate stress with certain challenging situations, such as examinations, job interviews, childbirth, an overwhelming workload, running a household, or coping with a range of complex feelings before undergoing surgery.

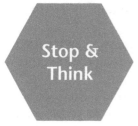

Think of specific situations which cause you stress. Are there clear patterns you can identify? Are there specific situations which you know trigger stress for you? Is there something particular about the experience which leads you to define it as stressful?

Factors that cause stress

Stress is caused by both internal and external factors – what we call stressors. The external factors that cause stress are usually associated with everyday life and can range from seemingly minor situations, such as not being able to find a car parking space, to highly significant experiences such as a bereavement or a threat to our safety. While some may be unwelcome, these situations or challenges abound, and arguably constitute normal life experiences – but their effect on us may be to produce feelings of stress.

The internal factors that cause stress may not be apparent or visible to other people and can stem from our thoughts, feelings or beliefs, whether or not they relate to particular situations. Internal stress may be triggered by feelings of uncertainty, pressure to cope or succeed, a fear that we may embarrass or shame ourselves in some way, expectations which exceed (or which we feel exceed) our ability, a feeling or perception that we lack the resources to deal with a situation, or perhaps low self-esteem. We want to underline that these are all extremely common and reflect states of being, and not mental illness. Everyone experiences feelings like this from time to time and in a range of situations.

The impact of internal or external sources of stress, however, differs from person to person. You will recognize particular situations or contexts which commonly produce stress for you. These are most likely to be the workplace, certain times during family interaction (such as mealtimes, preparing to go on holiday, or just trying to get things done), and being called on to perform in front of others, for example when being interviewed for a job, giving a speech or hosting a party.

Here are some reasons for people's different responses to stress:

1 We do not all interpret situations in the same way, and therefore while for one person a situation may be stressful, for another it may be a positive and welcome challenge.
2 Different people employ different skills in order to cope with challenging situations. If someone uses a personal coping mechanism easily and well, the situation does not then become stressful. (If someone has a coping skill but for some reason fails to employ it effectively, this may actually lead to an increase in the stress generated by the original situation.)
3 Where a source of stress is seen as being within your control you are more likely to be able to deal with the situation and manage the stress; where the source is not under your control this will not be the case.
4 Genetic make-up and family experience may predispose how people cope with stress.
5 There may be related factors which affect people's ability to cope with stress. For example, if you are feeling depressed when encountering a stressful situation, then the stress engendered by that situation will be more difficult to deal with and you may feel overwhelmed.

6 Similarly, if someone uses alcohol or recreational drugs in order to alleviate feelings of stress, this can actually intensify the feelings of stress and make the situation worse (hangovers do not help our coping mechanisms or enable us to see situations in an optimistic light, for example!).

Let's now look in a bit more detail at some of the ways in which stress can affect us.

How stress affects our emotions

Emotions or feelings are internal behaviours or reactions which most of us experience almost continuously while we are awake. Some of these emotions or feelings may be more prominent than others, and can be unwelcome when we associate them with stress. The following are feelings we typically associate with stress:

- tension and restlessness
- increased agitation
- sadness or low mood
- irritability
- anxious thoughts
- low self-confidence
- a tendency to become distracted, difficulty concentrating
- fearfulness
- difficulty making decisions
- lack of interest in life
- withdrawal from others
- loss of creativity
- isolation and loneliness
- increased frustration
- periods of confusion
- tearfulness.

Behavioural symptoms of stress

Most people who feel stressed come to recognize that, in addition to making them feel different from how they normally feel, their state can affect how they behave. Common patterns of behaviour related to stress include:

- changes in sleep patterns
- avoiding problematic situations
- difficulty in communicating with others
- procrastination, particularly with regard to challenging tasks
- changes in habits
- use of alcohol or recreational drugs, abuse of prescribed medications, etc.
- reliance on self-medication, such as for sleep and anxiety
- teeth grinding (bruxism)
- nail biting
- making excuses
- neglect of physical appearance
- loss of temper
- overreacting to situations
- seeming constantly rushed.

The body's stress alerts

There are also numerous physical signs and symptoms associated with stress. It is important to recognize that not all these signs and symptoms indicate that you are suffering from stress – they can also be present in other conditions. However, the following, particularly where several occur together, are likely to signal that you are experiencing stress:

- constantly increased heart rate
- muscular aches, pains and tension
- frequent headaches and backaches
- sweating, particularly in the palms and on the forehead
- sleep disruption
- dry mouth
- nausea and dizziness
- indigestion, stomach ache, heartburn, acid reflux, constipation or diarrhoea
- fluctuating weight

- skin problems (dryness, rashes, eczema, etc.)
- changes in breathing, including short, shallow breathing or frequent sighing.

Diana, a financial analyst in the City, had a heavy workload which led her to work late most evenings for a period of months. Although she was sleeping badly and felt her muscles constantly aching, she stopped exercising and seeing friends because she was spending so much time at work. In the office one evening she felt a sharp pain in her chest and thought she was having a heart attack; she asked her PA to call a cab and went straight to A&E. Examinations and tests came up negative and Diana was told she should rest. She went straight back to work and continued to work long hours each day. Her 'heart attack' symptoms occurred again, with increasing frequency (every time she felt stressed, adrenaline would be released in her body, leading to physical changes). She saw two private specialists for further investigations, but all tests continued to come back negative for heart and brain problems. Finally, on the advice of a third specialist, Diana went to see a psychologist who diagnosed stress.

Had Diana maintained her original lifestyle, which included exercise, socializing and relatively reasonable work hours, she would not have had the stress of thinking she had something medically very wrong with her and would have avoided a highly stressful visit to A&E and subsequent visits to medical professionals, not to mention a course of medication to deal with her stress. She ignored the early alerts her body gave her in warning (sleeping badly, unexplained aches and pains, etc.) because she would not take the time to attend to them – and in the end she spent more time dealing with them and exacerbated her stress problem.

Effects on thinking

As mentioned previously, our internal thoughts can give rise to stress or may reflect that we are in a stressed state. These thoughts commonly include self-statements such as:

- 'I can't do this'
- 'I won't manage to get this done in time'
- 'I won't be able to do this properly/satisfactorily'

- 'I'll be caught out'
- 'This is going to turn out badly'
- 'I'm going to fall flat on my face here'
- 'I can't cope with all this – there's just too much'
- 'I don't know where to begin'
- 'This will all end in disaster'

You will probably identify with at least a few, if not many, of the behavioural, emotional, physical and psychological symptoms of stress listed above. Even if you are fortunate enough not to be experiencing stress right now, it is likely that you recognize many of the symptoms from other times in your life when you *were* feeling stressed. It may be that you are more affected by physical symptoms of stress than behavioural ones. Or, by contrast, perhaps for you stress comes from internal thoughts and feelings but you do not display any outward signs.

One of the well-recognized aspects of stress is that it can be regarded as a low-grade toxic feeling, which can stop you from thinking clearly and getting on top of what is causing your stress. That is why there is a strong risk of stress becoming cumulative.

Prolonged or intermittent?

Does stress have to last for a prolonged period in order for you to class yourself as being stressed? This is a good and important question. It is possible to experience stress intermittently, for example at various points during each day or from time to time during the course of your life. Stress comes and goes, waxes and wanes. You may recognize stress at a time when you are particularly challenged, and then notice that you are no longer stressed once that challenge is out of the way. A typical example is someone waiting for the results of an examination: it is normal to feel stressed in advance because the result is unknown and you worry about how you have performed. Once you know the result – and the news is good – your stress levels subside. However, even if the news is bad your stress levels may go down because the uncertainty is now resolved and you can move on and make plans to deal with not having achieved the results you wanted.

Stress can also be associated with certain activities in a particular day. For example, people who commute, particularly in busy cities, usually feel stressed about congestion, delays and other travel problems. Delays increase physical stress, which in turn can give rise to more signs of stress. This stress may then abate or lift completely on arrival at work, until the next day when the commute has to be faced again.

Prolonged stress may be associated with normal life changes. During pregnancy, for example, some people feel stressed about starting or expanding a family. They may also be stressed about being away from work, the effect of the pregnancy on their relationship with their partner, giving birth, or whether or not the baby will be healthy.

Stress can arise out of traumatic situations such as serious illness, abuse or violent crime. Traumatic stress usually comes from situations where the event was not anticipated, and where we are unable to influence or control what happens. Some of the feelings experienced after such events, such as shame or anger, are also outside our control and trying to deal with these can be another great source of stress.

Many patients who require prolonged treatment for a medical condition, such as those undergoing chemotherapy for cancer or taking antiretroviral drugs for HIV, may feel stressed throughout the duration of their treatment, wondering about the outcome of the treatment and what the aftermath of the illness will mean for their lives – or even whether they are going to survive. They may also experience stress when actually taking medication or undergoing treatment, as some aspects of these may in themselves be unpleasant. A course of chemotherapy, for example, may involve unwelcome symptoms such as nausea, fatigue and lethargy.

It is important here too to recognize that stress is a part of life and should not in itself be viewed as a psychological problem or disorder which has to be treated or cured. Stress often indicates, rather than personal failure, difficulties in managing our lives. If addressed and managed well, stress can help us to gain confidence in our abilities, enabling us to acknowledge our personal limitations and to restore good physical and emotional health.

Myths about stress

At this point we would like to debunk some myths about stress. We hope this will reassure you about your own experience of it:

- Stress is not caused by any personal shortcoming or personality defect, although how people deal with life generally – and with stress specifically – may reflect their unique personality (we say more about this in the next chapter).
- Experiencing stress does not reflect on your intelligence or achievements.
- Stress is not the same for everyone: research has demonstrated that some personality types are more susceptible to stress, particularly those who have a tendency to anxiety or neurosis, or who demand overly high standards of themselves and others.
- Stress is not invariable: some people experience it more frequently than others and similar situations produce different stress reactions in different people.
- In most cases there is no way to predict whether someone will experience stress in a given situation.
- Stress is not inherently bad and can have positive effects (such as helping us to focus and to achieve, upping our game) as well as negative ones.
- It is not inevitable that too much stress over too long a period will become unmanageable and, unless corrective action is taken, lead to more significant psychological problems.
- Taking on a load of extra work does not cure stress – in fact the opposite is likely to be true.

In this last case, while working harder or taking on more will not cure stress, it is likely that by learning to work more smartly and efficiently, and by taking regular breaks away from work, you will be able to manage stress much more usefully. (It may be a cynical view, but some people have told us that they think their employer has a vested interest in encouraging the myth that an increased workload overcomes stress!)

Whatever the source, it is important to learn how to prevent stress if it is a recurring feature in your life. This may involve major life changes (such as finding a new job or career, or distancing a friend or family member), but if these changes are necessary to prevent recurrent and cumulative stress it is important that they should be identified and addressed.

It is virtually impossible to assess our stress levels at every moment in our lives. This would slow us down to a point where it became difficult to function normally. And, to repeat, stress is good – or at least acceptable – as long as we are in control and in charge of what is going on in our lives. What is important is to take regular stock, to reflect on and measure your own stress levels and try to identify what is causing a heightened level of stress, and to take steps to prevent it from escalating. And one of the aims of this book is to help you become your own stress manager. So let's now go on to consider in more detail the causes of stress.

3

What causes and/or maintains stress?

In understanding what causes stress, and what keeps it going in us (maintains it), we need to look at both external and internal mechanisms. We started to do this in the previous chapter, and now we are going to explore these mechanisms a little more deeply.

As we have seen, external contributors to stress might include major life events such as work or relationship changes, financial difficulty or bereavement; internal contributors might be having a pessimistic outlook on life, holding unrealistic expectations, being unable to accept uncertainty, being a perfectionist or lacking in assertiveness.

Internal factors or personal characteristics can also be instrumental in influencing how an individual copes with stress, and can go some way to explaining why what causes stress for one individual may have little or no impact on another. In this chapter we shall begin to explore why some people are more sensitive to stress than others, and look at some of the psychological phenomena which can underlie stress.

We will also invite you to think about your lifestyle, your social support and your current strategies for dealing with stress. The idea behind this is to encourage you to start thinking about the way you yourself experience stress and any underlying problems that may be contributing to your feelings of stress.

Why are some people more sensitive than others to stress?

As we have already mentioned, some people are highly sensitive to stress while others are more resilient. Some individuals are prone to experiencing emotions such as anxiety, sadness, frustration, anger and fear with greater intensity when facing adversity. Others are simply much less inclined to experiencing negative emotions. Each of us, though, is a combination of personality traits, consisting of innate characteristics and the effects of the environment that shapes us over the course of our lives – and especially during our formative years.

There is an argument in most of the influential strands of psychology that the quality of early life experience is critical in contributing to the adults that we become. (For example, a great deal of research suggests that individuals who have experienced adversity at an early age may be more susceptible to developing depression.) Certainly, the way we think about life may play a role in our sensitivity to stress. People whose childhoods were difficult, characterized for example by punitive or aggressive parenting, may as a result develop negative beliefs about themselves, other people and the world, and these beliefs may be activated during periods of stress. On the other hand, people who in childhood experienced a nurturing environment consisting of loving, caring and validating parenting will have been helped to develop into confident adults who are better equipped to deal with adversity. This is no simple cause-and-effect relationship, because research has also shown that for some individuals adverse early life experience allows them to develop the ability to cope better with life's stressors – they arm themselves with a certain level of resilience. Either way, however, early life experience certainly plays a role in determining how individuals will cope with stress later on.

Our genetic make-up may play a role in whether we tend to be sensitive or resilient to stress. Neuroscience has helped us to examine and understand this through study of the role of the nervous system. On the molecular level, there is evidence that certain variants of a gene that regulates the neurotransmitter serotonin – the chemical linked to our feelings of well-being – may mediate an individual's response to feelings such as depression and our levels of stress sensitivity. Research has also shown that there may be an association between the neurotransmitter known as neuropeptide Y and levels of stress. Higher levels of neuropeptide Y have been found to decrease response to fear and may contribute significantly to recovery from post-traumatic stress disorder. People whose genes predispose them to produce lower levels of neuropeptide Y have been found to be more responsive to negative stimuli, and these people are also more likely to suffer from major depressive disorders.

So both environment and genes play a crucial role in how we handle the pressures that we come across in our everyday life. We are not (yet at least) able to be sure whether genes or early environmental conditions play a more important role. What we do know is that we are all individual, and our very own biological make-up and our early environment will both, in some way, colour the way that we interact with our later, adult, environment.

Psychological problems underlying stress

When thinking about your own current stress, it is important to be able to recognize not just the symptoms but also the underlying factors that may be perpetuating the problem, so that these may be addressed. When someone sees that their personal resources are outweighed by the demands or pressures placed on them, stress is very likely to be the result. Therefore, when your personal resources are depleted in any way as a result of an undercurrent of psychological difficulties, you are naturally more vulnerable to the symptoms of stress.

Any one of a number of emotional difficulties could be underlying your stress. These might include a negative mood state such as guilt, unexpressed anger, depression, anxiety, grief, unhappiness or frustration. Or a difficult life situation might be the cause; you may, for example, feel stuck in a position where you are unable to see a way out, such as feeling dissatisfied with your job or relationship, or being isolated and experiencing intense loneliness.

It is very common in our clinical work to see a complex matrix of depression, anxiety and stress. Teasing these apart can be complicated, as in many cases they are closely intertwined. For example, if someone is experiencing an enduring negative mood state, then it is highly likely that they will also be experiencing more stress than, say, someone who feels relatively positive about their life and who is more or less happy with their lot.

Depression itself may result from a complex combination of genes, childhood experience, thinking style and difficult life events. In itself, depression tends to impede our ability to cope with challenges, and even the more trivial daily challenges may prove difficult to manage for people who are struggling with depression.

The same is true the other way round: struggling with unrelenting stress increases the potential for the onset of depression (which is then often known as 'stress-induced depression'). Studies have shown that repeated exposure to stress may disrupt the release of serotonin, the chemical linked to feelings of well-being and happiness. Depleted levels of serotonin are in turn linked to depression.

There is a similar reinforcing relationship between anxiety and stress – and although this is a close relationship it is important not to confuse the two. Anxiety and stress are different states: anxiety is related to exaggerated fear and its symptoms are frequently physiological, whereas stress is more a combination of psychological and physical tension. Anxiety and stress are often, like stress and depression, interlinked in a 'vicious circle', with stress creating anxiety and anxiety driving stress.

Struggling with underlying difficulties therefore tends to reduce our capacity to cope in general, so that when we inevitably have to face the challenging aspects of life – such as an overload of work, an unpleasant environment or some type of conflict – with depleted levels of resilience, we find it much harder to deal with them.

Since stress can be thought of as the consequence of a feeling that external demands exceed the personal resources we have within ourselves, in order to address the stress that you are experiencing, it is therefore important first of all to identify any underlying emotional difficulties that could be intensifying your reactions to the new pressure in your life.

What about lifestyle?

We have already discussed how stress can serve a useful purpose for some people at some times, by helping them to get things done rather than avoid and procrastinate. It can even actually enhance performance! However, enduring stress is not a good thing. Most of us are vulnerable to the detrimental long-term effects of stress, yet it is very easy to fall into the trap of becoming victims of life-styles that put us under continuing stress – and many of us do fall. The creation of balance in our lives is vital if we are to ensure that we avoid the pitfalls of overload and potential burnout.

Joe works as a banker in an extremely competitive environment. He regularly does a seventy-hour week and appearances at work are very important, so putting in overtime is viewed as necessary. Joe is desperately keen to gain promotion in order to move up to a higher salary bracket, and also to gain greater status within the company. Although he has a wife and two young children, he rarely sees them during the week as he leaves home early and returns late. At weekends he is exhausted and finds it very difficult to summon the energy to spend quality time with his family. He is generally irritable, and minor occurrences make him feel disproportionately angry with both his wife and the children. He rarely exercises and no longer has any out-of-work interests. He has very little time for pleasure. Joe has a very poor work-life balance and could be at risk of burnout.

Janet is the mother of two teenagers aged 13 and 15. She is also looking after her elderly parents: her father recently had a heart attack and her frail mother is unable to cope. Her husband works full time and travels frequently for his job. Janet's siblings all live too far away to be involved in the daily care of their parents. She finds it very difficult to delegate tasks and takes on the full load of responsibility on her own, worrying that others will not manage to do what she does and to the same standard. She also worries incessantly about her parents' deteriorating health. She does not ask for or expect any input from anyone else and she generally has poor levels of support. Janet is carrying an overload of responsibilities.

Jack started his own business two years ago. In spite of initial difficulties, it is now beginning to grow and he is very committed to its success. He ploughs all of his time into developing the business, including weekends. He has not taken on any staff who would be able to relieve him of his responsibility for managing all aspects of the business. Again, Jack has very little balance in his life, with work consuming most of his waking hours. He has no pleasurable activity or creative outlet. By depriving himself of any break he is denying himself any opportunity to step back and re-evaluate his situation.

Time away from the normal routine of life allows individuals to re-evaluate priorities and look at life through an alternative perspective. It also allows time to just switch off, to unwind and relax. For Joe, Janet and Jack life is like a treadmill with no breaks, relaxation or time to wind down. For none of them is there any balance between work and pleasure.

When considering why you are reacting in certain ways and feeling intensified pressure, it is imperative that you take a good look at your life and consider whether it is top-heavy in work or responsibility. It is likely that a poor work–life balance is intensifying your stress.

Do I have adequate support?

It is vital to recognize your habitual response to increased levels of stress. Some people may respond by withdrawing quietly to attempt to find a solution to their difficulties, perhaps not wanting to worry or burden others. This strategy can be helpful in some cases, but more often than not our social networks may be better able to offer support. Humans are relational creatures and tend to spend many years cultivating personal and professional connections, establishing networks, and these are a valuable resource when we need help.

Belonging to support networks can be very valuable on both a practical and emotional level. Professional networks are likely to have suitable knowledge and experience to provide information to help us navigate the stressor we are facing. Personal networks of family and friends may be able to help by listening to us, showing they care about us, and being willing to support us in working through the predicament we face. The knowledge that people care can in itself be comforting during difficult times and can help us feel more secure when facing difficulties. It can also boost self-esteem by making us feel worthy and loved. Friends and family may also help by offering alternative perspectives to a problem so that we can approach it from a different angle. They may be able to share their own similar experiences, or recommend pointers for further support. Being able to reach out to those around us can therefore be an incredibly important strategy for addressing our levels of stress in the longer term.

What are your current strategies for dealing with stress?

As we go through life we tend to develop personal strategies for dealing with stress. However, our choices may not always be the healthiest ones.

In order to understand your own stress better, it is helpful to be able to identify how you react to it, what coping strategies you employ and whether these are sufficient or whether they inadvertently contribute to escalating your stress levels.

Some people find themselves becoming dependent on alcohol after a long and pressurized day at work, to help them to unwind. For others, smoking cigarettes may help release tension. Some people turn to television or computer screens for their escapism from the realities of life. For yet others, food might offer the comfort that is so desperately craved when we feel overwhelmed.

Then there is avoidance, whereby procrastination or chronic oversleeping can offer a temporary escape from external pressures. Or, as we mentioned earlier, withdrawal from friends and family might seem to offer a space in isolation from the world, one in which we can avoid discussing our thoughts and feelings. For some people, denial can temporarily seem to offer protection from harsh reality and they simply refuse to acknowledge the symptoms of stress.

Needless to say, the above methods for coping with stress can be detrimental to our health in the longer term – and certainly avoidance and a reluctance to bite the bullet and tackle the issues that we face can lead to increased pressure rather than solving the source of stress. These are what we call 'flawed solutions'; people adopt them because they are easy, near to hand and involve little effort. The downside is that they will not only fail to deal with the source of your stress but will have long-term negative effects into the bargain.

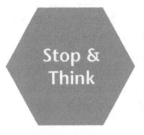

Stop & Think

What easy-to-turn-to habits have you adopted to help cope with your stress? Will these be harmful to you in the long term? How do you feel 'the morning after' – is your stress still there and do you feel unsatisfied, a sense of failure, 'I did it again'?

It is therefore important to think about your personal methods for coping and to consider how effective they are, and whether they are more harmful than helpful.

The stress-bucket approach

In order to examine your levels of vulnerability in relation to stress, it may be useful to use the analogy of the 'stress bucket'. As we said earlier in this chapter, we are all individual products of the complex matrices of our personal histories, the environments in which we live, and our genetic configuration. So we show varying degrees of tolerance for stress, and some people are far more resilient and able to cope, while others may feel much less able to deal with the pressure they face.

When you are faced with one stressful situation after another, think of them as a trickle of water dripping constantly into a bucket. Assuming the bucket has no hole in it, there is no way for the accumulating water to escape; it will eventually fill up and then overflow, unless you stop the dripping or empty the bucket. Stress works in a similar way. Essentially, if there is no outlet for the accumulating stress in you the chances are that, like the bucket, you will be unable to cope with the accumulation of negative feelings you are experiencing and you will be overwhelmed. And, as we discussed in Chapter 2, not moderating your stress is likely to put you at risk of a backlash of damaging psychological and physical symptoms.

If you are functioning healthily, then you are like a bucket with an outlet in it or leading from it, so the water never reaches the top and overflows. This helps to moderate the levels of stress experienced. If you are like this, you can accommodate the flow of stress through you, allowing space to successfully manage future stress.

In real-life terms, the outlet may come in the form of distraction, relaxation, escapism or pleasure and is essentially created through taking a much more balanced approach to life – unlike the people presented in the scenarios earlier in this chapter. We should always be mindful of making time for relaxation and fun; this then enables us to cope with life's stressors much more effectively. We should try to include relaxation time, connecting with others we care about, doing activities that we enjoy daily, and smiling and laughing, retaining some sense of humour even in the face of life's challenges and difficulties. Of course relaxation means different things to different people, but the starting point is giving yourself permission to do something pleasurable and relaxing for yourself, because greater balance is the key to a stress-reduced life! Below is a list of some simple activities aimed at helping us to relax:

- going for a walk, connecting with nature
- pottering in the garden
- visiting or calling a close friend or family member
- taking a long bath, with candles and scented oils
- treating yourself to a massage or otherwise pampering yourself
- listening to some of your favourite music
- watching an uplifting film
- going for a run or doing an intensive workout to relieve tension
- practising meditation
- interacting with pets
- doing or watching something amusing which makes you laugh.

The key is to figure out what helps you as an individual to relax – so experiment!

4

Why stress can be difficult to manage

What you need to manage your stress will of course depend on the type of person you are, your specific stressors, your circumstances, your personal resources, your personality, and your previous experience of stress. It will also depend on the choices you have in your life. In this chapter we will look at how you can replace ineffective coping strategies with more effective problem-solving to remove, reduce, reprioritize or accept sources of stress. Problem-solving techniques can be as diverse as reducing your workload, identifying when you need to say 'no' to people, or switching off your mobile phone at a set time each night.

We will also look further at the concept of 'flawed solutions' to dealing with stress, such as avoidance, alcohol and drug misuse, persistence, bargaining and blaming. These flawed solutions can get in the way of actually dealing with stress. The aim of this chapter is to help you identify more effective ways of dealing with stress.

Excessive stress is one of many psychological problems which require a holistic approach, looking at your whole lifestyle and finding ways suited to you and your personality by which you can build effective coping strategies. Tackling the problem of excessive stress also requires time, persistence and patience. However, we are (justifiably!) optimistic that almost everyone can learn to manage their stress.

James never thought he would be able to manage his load of stress. A couple of years ago his wife became ill and he was left combining a stressful job in the City with being the primary carer for their children. He tried to cope by cutting down on sleep because he felt there were never enough hours in the day. It was not long before he felt exhausted and became moody towards his colleagues and his children, and his performance at work deteriorated. James felt irritable, frustrated and often anxious. When his eldest son called James 'a ratty old fart', he decided to seek help for his stress. He contacted the confidential counselling service at work and, with their help, was able to prioritize his workload more effectively and realize the need for extra help at home.

Unhelpful coping strategies

You may have already tried some coping techniques and found that none of them have brought you closer to managing your stress. Some of the methods you have tried may have quelled your anxiety for a short period of time but, in the long term, simply masked the problem – or may even have made the effects of excessive stress worse.

Psychologists who work with people experiencing high levels of stress have recently turned their attention to what maintains stress, or keeps it going. This can be just as important as establishing what causes stress in the first place.

There are some common factors that can keep your stress levels high, and it is necessary to recognize these and understand, if they are part of your coping strategies, how they might affect you. Here are some examples of unhelpful strategies which people often use to cope with stress.

Procrastination Most people procrastinate at some point in their lives. This behaviour can cause stress in the first place, but it can also maintain or amplify symptoms of stress. A good example is when you are studying for an exam but keep putting off revising, constantly promising yourself 'It'll be better if I start after I've had some relaxation time' or 'People revise better when they do it at the last minute'. As you get closer to the day of the exam you feel increasingly stressed about the fact that you have not revised sufficiently. Another example of procrastination is to delay confronting pressing issues and instead spend time on less important matters ('displacement activity').

Catastrophizing Because stress can cause you to feel overwhelmed, it can seem that even small changes to your day or minor tasks are like 'having a big mountain to climb'. And when people feel overwhelmed they are more prone to make catastrophic interpretations of a situation, where they focus their attention on everything that might go wrong (as opposed to right).

Tom, a very good footballer, had recently lost his grandfather. This made him feel stressed, especially now that his grandmother was living by herself. During the lead-up to important games, Tom noticed that he spent a great deal of time thinking about all the possible things that could go wrong, including losing the game, playing badly and therefore losing his position in the team, or injuring himself. Whenever he had a minor argument with his girlfriend, Tom convinced himself that she was going to end their relationship. He was also very afraid that something awful would happen to his grandmother, such as falling down the stairs in her home or getting ill (despite the fact that she was in excellent health).

Catastrophic interpretations can make a situation seem much more frightening than it actually is, thus undermining your ability to deal with the situation.

Avoidance You may avoid confronting problems, situations, people or places with which you feel unable to cope. It is perfectly normal to try to avoid something that you think is dangerous, but if the situation is actually safe it may be more your anticipatory fear that prevents you from identifying and solving the problem.

Neil and Holly were experiencing marital difficulties. Holly was very keen to attend couples counselling as she felt this would allow them to confront the source of the escalated and stressful arguments they had at home. Neil, on the other hand, found it difficult to commit to couples sessions because he thought that they would be painful and frustrating.

Although it can be difficult to discuss emotionally charged topics, avoiding the situation is unlikely to help Neil and Holly solve their problems. In many cases, avoidance can make stress worse because it keeps you from realizing that you *can* cope with situations that you find stressful. If Neil, in the above example, had been prepared to attend marital therapy, he might have realized that he was capable of sharing his emotions with his wife. Avoidance can also result in a great loss of confidence which can affect how you feel about yourself.

Difficulties with saying 'no' Stress can drive us to behave in ways that we think will help us feel safe, or at least less stressed. Acting like this may not be helpful in the long run because it makes you feel even more stressed in other ways.

> Lisa was frequently asked by colleagues to take on additional tasks at work, despite being very busy with her own workload. She did not want colleagues to think of her as 'lazy' or 'unhelpful'. She stayed late in the office most days and would often bring work home. This made Lisa immediately feel less stressed about the prospect of being disliked by her colleagues. However, she eventually became exhausted and had to take time off from work to recover.

The problem was that Lisa never dared to say 'no' to her colleagues. She therefore did not get the chance to discover that most people would approve of her even if she refused to help out with their work. In the end she had to take time off work, which obviously impacted negatively on her colleagues anyway. Other common behaviours of this type include suppressing your own needs to please others, over-thinking social situations, and 'going overboard' to accommodate other people.

Excessive worry If you are spending too much time concentrating on your stress, you may actually be reinforcing it and reducing your capacity to do anything constructive to manage it. You may think that by worrying about stressful events you will be able to prevent them from happening. For example, you may 'catastrophize' (see above), imagining the worst that might happen prior to and during a stress-induced situation, and make a mental note of how to deal with each of these possible catastrophes. Catastrophizing and its subsequent thoughts can significantly increase your stress levels.

Blaming others It is sometimes easy to blame our stress on other people or on external circumstances. Have you ever thought to yourself that your life would be so much easier if your boss was more empathetic? Or what about the occasions when you've heard a friend say 'If the trains were more reliable I would have been on time'? Young people particularly have a wonderful way of blaming external objects for their own mistakes. A young child, for example, may bang his foot on the table and then ask his parents whether they can put the table on the naughty step because IT hurt his foot! This is true for adults too; sometimes it is unconscious, but at other times this blaming is a deliberate move to preserve dignity or to avoid taking responsibility. This strategy can also be used where someone simply does not feel they have the energy to change the circumstances or situation that is causing their stress.

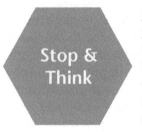

Stop & Think

To help you identify the degree to which you contribute to your stress, try asking yourself the following questions: To what degree do my actions or what I say contribute to the stress I'm feeling? Is there anything I can do to alleviate the source of my stress? Am I being defensive about the situation, or is it really due to other people/external circumstances?

Over-stretching Some people like to keep busy and therefore try to fit as much into their day as they possibly can. This may be because they are highly ambitious, or it may be fuelled by a need to balance many different roles and responsibilities. However, if you try to cope with life stressors and increased responsibilities by 'doing them all' – taking on too much over an extended period of time – stress and exhaustion can gradually build up until they become overwhelming.

> Alison combined a full-time post as a sister at a busy hospital with bringing up three young children and serving as a board member of a charity for homeless people. Her husband travelled a great deal with his work and was often abroad for long periods of time. There was rarely any time for Alison to relax or attend to her own needs.

> Alex, a young lawyer, was keen to become a partner in the law firm where he worked. He continuously strove to be noticed by working long hours and signing up for conferences and professional courses whenever he could. This left little time to engage in other activities and he gradually became increasingly stressed and isolated.

Although it is normal to keep busy during stressful periods at home or at work, over-stretching yourself over long periods of time can affect your physical and psychological health – and can often be counterproductive by reducing your ability to work effectively.

Excessive use of alcohol, recreational drugs, etc. Some people use alcohol to help them quell their nerves when they are feeling anxious or stressed. However, the stress often re-emerges soon afterwards as the effects of the alcohol wear off. Long term, there is obviously the potential to develop a new problem: over-reliance on alcohol. This over-reliance can lead people to think that their ability to endure stress-inducing situations is due to the use of alcohol rather than to other skills and techniques. (Incidentally, very occasionally some prescribed medications can increase stress and anxiety – so it is always advisable to check with your GP if this is the case for you.) Alcohol may seem to be a useful and easily available remedy for stress, but it does not help you to solve or overcome the problem. With smoking and recreational drugs, etc. – similarly unhelpful strategies – the story is the same.

Stop & Think

Are you able to assess your ability to cope? For example, are you blaming others, procrastinating or being avoidant? Note some of the things you have done or would do to deal with stress. If you are unsure, you can use this book to guide your awareness of potential coping strategies. Make a clear distinction between strategies that help you to deal with stress a bit better (for example assertiveness, confronting the source of your stress, etc.) and safety behaviours that prevent you from dealing with your stress (such as procrastination, blaming others, etc.). Select one unhelpful coping behaviour you would like to stop using.

Finding the resources to put these skills into practice

Motivational issues can also interfere with progress in reducing your stress level. We are not suggesting that if you struggle with excessive stress you do not really want to overcome it – this is unlikely to be the case. However, overcoming your stress problem requires time, focus and intensity. Are you firing on all these cylinders? If not, it may be because of the stress itself, or other difficulties in your life may be distracting you from dealing with the problem. In our experience, very few people have the luxury of working on their stress without having other issues, or multiple stressors, to deal with. It may be that you are having a difficult time at work, for example, or are stressed by a misbehaving child, or are facing health problems in the family.

Your motivation may also be affected by the fact that you have lived with stress and its symptoms for a long time. You may therefore have developed reasonable coping solutions whereby, again, you avoid or manage – rather than solve – the problem. Sometimes being comfortable with your own solution to the problem, even though it is not actually a solution but rather a coping strategy, can interfere with your efforts to overcome and cure the problem. Change is difficult at the best of times, so your motivation may naturally be more towards leaving things as they are than pushing on with change.

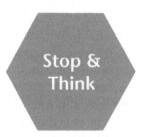

Stop & Think

Ask yourself a series of reflective questions to assess your circumstances and motivation, such as: Am I comfortable in my ways? Is it too much effort to make the necessary change? Do I have the energy, stamina or motivation to confront the source of my stress? Are the gains I could make outweighed by the comfort I feel staying as I am?

You might also consider whether anything else in your life is holding you back from making changes in your behaviour and dealing with uncomfortable and/or stressful feelings.

Bear in mind that dealing with stress requires time, patience, perseverance and a great deal of determination. There may be occasional setbacks, or it may feel as if you are playing a game of snakes and ladders: first progress is suddenly reversed, then the process quickly picks up steam again. Maintaining a positive outlook, a healthy dose of motivation, and keeping the ideas described in this book in mind, will help to keep you focused and on track.

It may help if you occasionally revisit your goals. You can use the following questions to guide the process of staying focused:

- Are your goals realistic (for example are they not too difficult, but not too easy either)?
- Is it possible to break your goal into a smaller set of sub-goals?
- Can you think of ways to measure your progress so that you can see it (for example, what are you able to do now that you were unable to do when you first started to work on your goal)?
- Have you allowed yourself enough time to achieve your goals?

Finding assistance

Involving others – whether friends and family or professionals – in your treatment and problem-solving can be enormously helpful. Of course, the act of talking to someone else about your problem may be the first and most obvious stumbling block. It may be embarrassing or stressful even to describe the problem to another person – who may not even be aware of it in the first place. Also, bringing yourself into close emotional proximity to others is something many people find difficult. We would however encourage you to do this because trained and experienced specialists in this area will have encountered many people with similar problems. For them, the problem will not be new and nor will it be an uncomfortable situation. On the contrary, it is their job to help you with this difficulty and they should give you every encouragement along the way. Your stress problem is a treatable psychological condition, so you can expect support and help in your efforts to overcome it.

If you take the problem to a trained professional, your starting point at your first meeting could be that you have recently read a book on overcoming stress (this one!) and, on the basis of what you have read, you think you might be suffering from excessive stress. If you have been able to apply some of the ideas you have learnt in the book, you may also be able to describe why and how you feel the problem has come about and what you have done so far in order to overcome it. You could also describe why you feel you are not making adequate progress in reducing your stress.

We recognize that taking the problem to someone else means facing up to it and putting it in words to another person. Think of it as part of your therapy, because describing the problem and talking about it with another person is in itself therapeutic. Describing our problems is a major way in which we learn more about how they affect us and how we feel about them. It is an important first step in bringing about change.

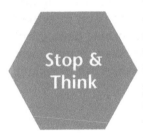

Is there anyone you can think of whom you would find it relatively easy to talk to (for example a friend, family member, colleague or teacher)? When would be the best time for you to talk to someone else about the issues you are experiencing? What would you essentially want the other person to do (just listen, offer practical advice on how to manage your stress, offer empathy and understanding, help you to find a psychologist, therapist or counsellor)?

A session with your GP, psychologist, counsellor or therapist will help to put you back on track by assessing the nature and extent of your problem and how to treat it. This book can then act as a companion to that face-to-face treatment, and you can use the book to help you think about homework exercises and in plotting your progress.

5

How to build resilience in the face of stress

By this stage in the book you will have realized that managing your stress requires working with what you do and what you think, as well as learning to identify and deal with the source of your stress.

Finding a new way of doing something can often be highly effective – so looking at breaking your unique cycle of stress differently may well work for you. This chapter explores practical ways of trying out new behaviours and building your confidence in order to manage your stress. We will describe the techniques most likely to work for you in managing stress. These include dealing with procrastination, becoming more assertive, sleep management, learning to organize and prioritize tasks to reduce over-stretching, physical exercise, and learning to relax.

Monitoring progress

Using the information you have already collected as you have worked through this book, you will have a good chance of choosing a technique which is likely to be effective for you. Nobody, however – and certainly not psychologists! – gets it right first time, every time. That is why it is so important to monitor the techniques you select, and not invest too much time and effort trying to make a solution work if it is not effective for you.

When you have chosen a technique to help manage your own stress, read the description of that technique again and make sure that you understand why you have chosen that particular one, why it may be helpful for you, and what it involves.

Sharing some of the work you are doing with a trusted friend or family member can be enormously helpful. If you have someone helping you, a good way of checking that you understand the technique is to try and explain to them what it is and why you have chosen it. If you can do that, you can be confident that you understand what you are doing.

Once you understand why you have chosen to try a particular technique, it is equally important to monitor your progress to check that you are actually achieving what you set out to achieve. Here are some suggested ways you can do this:

- Give your feeling of stress a score of 0 to 10, where 0 is feeling perfectly calm and 10 refers to maximum stress level. When you are in situations which have triggered stress for you in the past, make a note of your score. If the techniques you are using are effective, your score will reduce over time.
- Keep a tally of the number of times you do things that either help manage your stress or contribute to it. If the technique you have chosen is working for you, unhelpful behaviours will reduce and helpful ones will increase.
- Set a sensible goal and plan a reward for when you achieve it.

Techniques for managing stress

The techniques suggested in the following pages are by no means an exhaustive list of ways to manage your stress. As we have said before, each person's stress is essentially unique, so it is therefore important that you identify what you personally need in order to manage your stress better. You may find that the source of your stress is at the organizational level at work, in which case talking to management, human resources, or even getting a business coach may be a possible solution. If you are struggling with your home life you may want to think about the resources you need to help you cope, such as domestic help, childcare or marital counselling. Whatever your situation, however, we hope that the methods we describe will help you become more efficient at dealing with the source of your stress, as well as helping you to build resilience so that you become less affected by it.

Dealing with procrastination

Everyone procrastinates at some point in their lives. However, prolonged episodes of procrastination can be particularly unhelpful because they may prevent you from returning to the task you were postponing. During such episodes the number of tasks will gradually accumulate. Before you know it, there will be a whole heap of things waiting to be done. If you continue to put things off, or you tend to do them at the very last minute, this may cause you a great deal of stress. In this situation, a vicious circle can be created, leading you to procrastinate further because even the smallest tasks come to seem overwhelming. This vicious circle of procrastination and stress can have a negative impact on your mood and your general well-being.

Consider trying the following to reduce procrastination:

1 Identify the tasks, situations or people likely to trigger procrastination. Then actively resist the trap of starting to procrastinate by prioritizing the jobs that you are most likely to keep putting off ('Do feared things first'). Completing the first difficult job successfully will help motivate you to start the next one, and each subsequent task will become easier as your sense of achievement and satisfaction grows.
2 Set aside time to confront procrastination. Schedule a specific time, day and place where you can deal with the situations you want to put off. Set an alarm to remind yourself.
3 Reduce or remove distractions so you can concentrate on the task you have been putting off. This may include switching off your mobile phone, letting people know you are unavailable for a certain period of time, delegating other jobs, etc.
4 Be organized. Try to think of the resources you need to complete the task.
5 If you encounter obstacles while tackling procrastination, think of ways to overcome these. Use problem-solving whenever necessary – try to identify what is holding you up and find a suitable solution that will enable you to move on from the obstacle – as this will reduce the risk of giving in to the temptation of giving up and procrastinating even more.

6 Recognize the efforts you are making to deal with procrastination. Give yourself a (short!) break between each task you complete. Use the break to reward yourself with a small treat.

Being assertive

All of us, at some point in our lives, find it difficult to deal with certain situations: saying 'no' to a friend, family member or colleague, standing your ground when someone is being aggressive or hostile towards you, pointing out to someone that they are acting unreasonably, for example. If we deal with these situations by saying nothing, or by becoming aggressive, we may experience feelings of stress or lose confidence in our ability to handle challenging situations.

Being assertive is not the same as being aggressive, rude or inconsiderate of other people's wishes or preferences. Assertiveness means communicating your feelings, intentions or opinions in a clear but non-aggressive and non-confrontational way.

Yvonne was in charge of the parent committee at the local primary school her daughter attended. She had a background in business and management but had given up her career when her daughter was born. She enjoyed being involved at her daughter's school and dedicated most of her spare time to organizing fundraising events and helping out with school activities. A majority of the parents whose children attended the school really appreciated Yvonne's efforts. However, during the monthly parental meeting one of the other mothers accused Yvonne of taking on too many tasks, which prevented other parents getting involved. Initially Yvonne felt upset and stressed about the remark. She contemplated stepping down from her position as the head of the committee, thinking that this would enable other parents to take more responsibility. However, she decided instead to email all the parents asking for volunteers to take over some of the jobs she was currently doing. Apart from a couple of parents who were already involved with the school, most responded that they didn't have the time to volunteer. During the next monthly parental meeting, Yvonne plucked up the courage to speak to the woman who had made the original remark, offering her the chance to volunteer. The woman hesitantly told Yvonne that she was not able to do this because she was a working mother. In a calm and friendly manner, Yvonne replied that she would welcome her involvement should she have time in the future.

If Yvonne had resigned from the committee without asking the other parents to become more involved, she may have thought the original remark to be true. This may well have caused her to feel stressed, and to worry that other people saw her as bossy and pushy. Instead she was assertive in letting the woman who had challenged her know that she disagreed with her remark.

You will find a range of assertiveness techniques in Chapter 10.

Dealing with sleep problems

From time to time, many people have problems sleeping. The amount of sleep each individual needs varies, and your sleep requirements will change throughout your life. As a general guideline, babies and young children need more sleep than adults and most older people need less sleep than at any other time in their lives. The normal range of sleep for an adult is anything between six and ten hours per night.

Difficulties with sleeping can be caused by psychological problems such as depression or anxiety. They can also be caused by stress, whether at work or in relationships. The problem is not only that stress can cause sleep problems, but that sleep problems can also amplify stress – so here is another vicious circle. You may for example notice that you worry more about sleep if you are finding it difficult to sleep and the worrying, in turn, may prevent you from sleeping because you are releasing adrenaline into your body. Adrenaline revs up your body for fight or flight – it certainly does not prepare you for sleep!

> Emily was revising for her final exams at university when she began to suffer sleep problems. She often stayed up until the small hours trying to revise as much as possible, which left her feeling tired the next day. When she tried to go to bed earlier in the evening, she couldn't sleep because her mind was racing with worry about the exams. She felt increasingly stressed about not getting enough sleep, which prevented her from studying efficiently. Three days before her first exam Emily went to see her GP, who recognized that Emily was stressed and sleep deprived. She was given helpful tips on how to manage her sleep as well as a light sleep medication to ensure that she got some rest before her exams.

Sleep disruption can have a negative impact on the way you think, feel and act. It is therefore important that you try, to the best of your ability, to maintain healthy sleep patterns during periods of stress. We give you some tips for dealing with sleep problems in Chapter 10. If you are finding it difficult to switch off your mind at night, you may also find the next chapter on dealing with stressful thoughts and worry helpful. It is important, of course, if you think that your sleep problems might have a physical cause, to check this with your GP – but use the tips in Chapter 10 rather than resorting to sleep medication if there is nothing physically wrong with you, because sleep medication is only a short-term solution.

Learning to organize and prioritize tasks

You probably remember a time when you felt overwhelmed by the things you had to do on a particular day or during a particular week. Have you ever wished there were more than 24 hours in the day so you could get everything done?

How do you find time to deal with everything you have to do in your life without falling into the trap of becoming excessively stressed, run down or tired? Most people, regardless of their individual background and resources, are restricted by time limitations and are consequently prone to periods of doing too much or overstretching themselves. This can cause stress, emotional and physical tiredness, as well as exhaustion. It is therefore important to organize your day effectively so that you can achieve most of the things you want and need to do.

The key is to 'work smart, not hard'. As there really are only 24 hours in each day, it is essential to plan so that your time does not just 'disappear' and you do not become frustrated and stressed by feeling at the end of each day that you have completed only a little of what you wanted, or needed, to achieve. There are some useful tips and hints in Chapter 10 to help you start to organize your life, and it is well worth while hunting out a book on the subject. Many such books are available, and one of them will be right for you.

Physical exercise

Another way to become more relaxed is to engage in regular exercise. Exercise helps your body to relieve the tension caused by stress. Exercise does not have to be over-strenuous or 'military' in style – it can include going for a brisk walk, or even just walking up a set of stairs as opposed to taking the lift or escalator. If you enjoy more strenuous exercise, then going to the gym, for example, might be fun and rewarding for you – but if not, then taking up a social hobby which involves vigorous exercise (such as dancing, tennis or swimming) is another option.

These are among the benefits of regular exercise:

- It has a positive effect on your mood. Exercise stimulates various chemicals in our bodies, such as endorphins, which leaves us feeling happier and more relaxed.
- It stimulates blood flow, oxygen and nutrient use in your body and helps your entire cardiovascular system work more efficiently.
- It can help you fall asleep faster and deepen your sleep.
- It has a positive effect on your health, weight and energy levels.

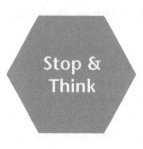

Stop &
Think

What type of physical exercise do you think you could do, or might enjoy (for example walking, jogging, cycling, dancing, climbing)? Think about a time of the day and the week when it would be easiest for you to start exercising. What is stopping you from doing physical exercise (health concerns, lack of time, lack of motivation, fear of looking or feeling stupid, needing to buy the necessary equipment or clothing, etc.)? Try to think about ways to overcome these obstacles and implement your solutions accordingly (for example getting health clearance from your GP, or joining a dance class with a friend to increase your motivation and enjoyment).

You can start exercising by setting yourself small goals such as walking instead of driving whenever possible, signing up for a gym or for dance classes, or digging your bicycle out of the garage and trying it out again.

Learning to relax

Learning relaxation skills is a vital part of treating stress because it helps you to manage the physical symptoms caused by stress. These skills will help you gain a sense of control over your unpleasant sensations and thoughts, and enable you to feel more confident emotionally. Becoming proficient in relaxation techniques will also show you that you *can* cope with difficult situations.

Controlling the physical symptoms of stress is a technique which needs to be practised frequently before you can expect to gain mastery and obtain lasting benefits. It is just like learning to drive: you need to keep practising until you are able to co-ordinate the many skills required without consciously thinking about them. It can be a challenge at first, especially when trying to apply relaxation skills in a difficult situation. It is therefore important to start by practising in settings where you feel comfortable and less stressed.

Slowing down your breathing

Using the breathing technique explained in Chapter 10, you can learn to relax through breathing. The technique is easy to apply and will help to reduce tension, anxiety and stress; it basically involves taking gentle, even breaths which fill your lungs completely, and then exhaling slowly. Deep breathing releases tension in your body and relaxes you; it is impossible to feel strained or stressed while you are concentrating on your breathing and controlling it, so practising this technique provides real 'time out'. (It also gives your brain and body an oxygen boost, which helps concentration and energy levels, among other benefits.)

You may find it a challenge to practise controlled breathing at first. You may feel as if you are not getting enough air or that the pace of your breathing seems unnaturally slow. This is a normal reaction when you practise a new routine. As your skill improves and you learn to relax quickly, you will find it easier to switch to correct breathing whenever you feel stressed.

You may want to progress to practising your breathing technique in more distracting situations and with your eyes open, for example while caught in a traffic jam or waiting outside the school gates to collect the children. The technique is simple and can be used at any stage of a stressful experience to reduce the likelihood of cumulative stress.

Releasing physical tension

Once you have learned the skill of relaxing your muscles, your mind and body will automatically feel calmer. However, the ability to relax physically does not always come easily; like correct breathing, it is a skill that needs to be learnt gradually and practised regularly. As we have seen, stress is different for each of us. We may not have the same bodily symptoms; each of us has our own independent stressful thoughts and each of us behaves differently when under stress. It is therefore important to find a relaxation technique that works for you. This is best done by practising the technique regularly before you use it in a stressful situation, so that you get used to doing it and gain confidence in its benefits.

In Chapter 10 you will find an exercise for progressive muscular relaxation. This exercise will teach you to recognize tenseness in your muscles and allow you to learn to control the tension in your body, which is a key method of reducing bodily stress – and if your body is relaxed it is very difficult for your mind to be stressed!

Setting goals

Goal-setting is an important and useful contribution to making the techniques in this chapter work for you. If, however, you set yourself a goal which is too difficult to reach, or one where it would be hard to know if or when you had achieved it, this will simply add to your difficulties.

There are specific strategies for goal-setting. Rather than just formulating a vague goal in your head ('I should stop getting so stressed by things at work') or simply making a resolution ('I'm going to get less stressed at work') – even one that includes a timed element ('Right, it's a new year now, and by the end of it I'm going to be less stressed at work') – you need to be precise in formulating what you want to achieve, how you are going to achieve it, how you are going to evaluate your progress along the way towards your goal, and in what timescale you are going to achieve it. In Chapter 10 we describe in detail the technique known as SMART goal-setting. Using this strategy in formulating your goals will give you the best chance of managing your stress.

This chapter has introduced you to the most important ways of actively reducing stress by learning new ways to cope with its sources. We would recommend that you try them all (relaxation techniques, assertiveness skills, prioritization and sleep management) in order to find out which ones work best in building your resilience and preventing you from being affected by excessive stress.

6

How to manage your thoughts and emotions during stress

It is likely that there are a number of different components involved in your experience of stress. In particular, though, the quality of your thoughts and emotions are likely to be a major driver or maintenance factor.

Thoughts have a significant impact on the way we feel in relation to certain events or situations and, as discussed earlier, perception plays a significant role in influencing the way we feel. For example, if your neighbour passes you on the other side of the road, not making eye contact with you and looking down all the time, what do you make of that? You might think she is trying to avoid you because she can't be bothered with you, or even doesn't particularly like you, and this may trigger a spiral of negative thinking about yourself. On the other hand, you might think she was just preoccupied and perhaps had something serious on her mind. This might make you feel concerned about her and want to know what is wrong – and perhaps you will call round at her house later and see if you can help. The neighbour is acting in exactly the same way in each scenario – but the *thinking*, the *perception*, has led to two very different interpretations of the same event.

Twenty-year-old Marie was brought to counselling by her father. The family were constantly arguing with one another and some of the arguments had become quite physical. Family interaction had become toxic, to the point where Marie and her father were living in the family's flat in the West End of London, and Marie's mother and siblings were living in their house in the country. Marie's father said that the really bad arguments always seemed to start when Marie reacted strongly and negatively to neutral things which members of the family said, but when she was not around there were no toxic arguments. When her father left, Marie recounted how she was the 'odd one out', both in the family and at school, where she had been excluded from the various friendship groups and cliques, and said the same thing was happening in the college where she was currently taking a modelling and secretarial course. She recounted an incident when she was young where she heard her mother and father discussing her, with her mother saying 'Marie is different, she's not like the rest of us.' Marie said that she knew everyone thought that about her, she could tell by the way they reacted. Just then, the practice receptionist came into the room and, excusing herself to Marie, whispered to me that my partner was on the phone and it was an emergency. I left the room to take the call and, when I returned, Marie was aggressive and hostile and soon terminated the session.

In a later session Marie said, 'Your receptionist thinks I'm odd too – I could see what she was thinking that day when she came in and she looked at me all the time when she was whispering to you about me.' I called in the receptionist and asked her to recall that day. She said, 'Oh yes, the day your mother was taken into hospital and your partner called – I remember [turning to Marie] that you were here and you were wearing that fabulous Dolce & Gabbana trouser suit and it looked so good on you – I was really jealous.'

From a single remark, which her parents did not even remember and which related to one particular incident (Marie's mother wondered if it might have related to a family game which Marie always won because she took a different, unexpected approach from the rest of the family), Marie's view of people around her had become distorted. She always interpreted their actions towards her in one way: they thought she was odd. This caused her to react to new acquaintances and complete strangers with hostility, and to attack as a form of defence and deflection.

Common thinking errors

When we are feeling stressed we may have exaggerated, distorted or unpleasant thoughts and feelings about things or situations. These thoughts tend to be negative and reflect our concerns about how and why we might not be able to cope. They range from mild apprehension, such as 'I'm not sure that I'm going to cope very well with being a parent', to extreme fears, such as 'My career is over if I don't do well in this new job'. These feelings can dent our confidence, lower our mood and make us feel negative, vulnerable, depressed, even out of control. Psychologists have identified a number of common thought patterns that reflect and maintain negative emotions. The most common ones are:

- *All-or-nothing thinking*: a tendency to think in absolute or extreme terms (also known as 'black-and-white thinking') about a situation, mostly in a negative way. For example: 'I could never be a successful person, I'm not good at anything.'
- *Over-generalization*: taking an individual case and making it apply in general terms. For example: Because you didn't sell many cakes at the school fête, you can never be involved in helping your child's school raise money in future. This discounts other relevant information, such as the fact that it was a rainy day and not many people attended the fête in the first place.
- *Mental filter*: focusing on negative or upsetting experiences or thoughts while ignoring other aspects that paint a different picture of the situation. For example: 'Moving home is too stressful and upsets the whole family.' The reality is that, even though the move itself was stressful, your family settled into the new home quite quickly and your partner and children are flourishing in the new surroundings, but this important information is ignored or discounted.
- *Disqualifying the positive*: discounting positive experiences as if you do not want to validate them, or being unable to replace your strongly held pessimistic view of life with anything more positive. For example: 'I know I've got a close relationship with my partner, but we always get into conflict whenever we come up against challenges.'
- *Jumping to conclusions or mind reading*: a tendency to assume that the worst will happen in spite of a lack of evidence to support that assumption. For example: 'I'm not going to get this job – the second interviewer didn't like me' – despite the fact that you know nothing about the interviewer and her normal way of reacting in an interview situation.
- *Catastrophizing*: interpreting the characteristics of a person or aspects of a situation negatively and in an exaggerated way, and foreseeing very bad consequences as a result, however unlikely.

For example: 'My boss is always cool towards me and never friendly, which has got to mean he doesn't like me or he thinks my work isn't good enough – I'm going to get sacked!'

- *Emotional reasoning*: making decisions based on how you feel rather than on facts and realities. For example: 'I'm not going to make an offer for that house although it seems perfect – that old teddy bear left in the cellar really freaked me out.'
- *'Should', 'must' and 'have to'*: when your thoughts are somehow distorted, which tends to 'fix' you rigidly in a situation and makes it seem that you are governed by inflexible or extreme rules. For example: 'I should be able to cope with this. I shouldn't have all these unpleasant feelings. It must be because the pills aren't working. I'll have to give up my job.' (A famous therapist called Albert Ellis rather wickedly termed this tendency 'musterbation'!)
- *Labelling and mislabelling*: putting a label (usually negative) on someone, or on yourself, based on just one characteristic personality trait. Specifically, 'mislabelling' is putting a negative 'spin' on a person, for example labelling yourself 'sexually unattractive' because your first partner left you for someone of the same sex as themselves. Or you might mislabel someone who sends their child to boarding school as 'a selfish parent' because you personally think that childhood should be spent at home.
- *Personalization and blame*: exaggerating causation when the facts do not necessarily support your interpretation ('taking things personally'). For example: 'I got to Auntie Linda's house and she started shouting at me as soon as I walked in the door – I must have done something really wrong', when in fact Auntie Linda was in a bad mood which had no connection with your arrival.

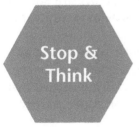

Stop & Think

Read through the above thinking errors one more time. See if you can recognize any of them among your own thought processes. Make a note of your thoughts. Are you able to link your individual thoughts to any or all of the ten common thinking errors?

Managing negative thoughts

It is crucial to recognize the role of thought and perception as drivers for the emotions that we experience, and in our whole view of the world. If you have constant worrying thoughts in relation to the stress you are feeling, these will add to your stress symptoms. The stress can then inadvertently lead to a range of unpleasant and overwhelming feelings such as anger, irritability, despair, anxiety, fear and hopelessness.

Feeling overwhelmed by uncomfortable and negative emotions can be frightening, and may hamper your ability to see a solution or a way forward. What's more, this feeling of being overwhelmed may have a broader impact by preventing you from focusing or concentrating properly on anything. It may harm relationships by stopping you from being able to interact without becoming irritable or angry, and may generally get in the way of your daily life and functioning.

Ultimately, trying to deal with a tidal wave of negative emotions prevents us from being able to experience pleasure and enjoy life. Powerful negative emotions can feed off one another and lead to further physical, cognitive and behavioural symptoms of stress.

What follows are a range of techniques to help you approach and better manage the negative feeling states or emotions you experience as a result of stress. These require just a little effort and commitment. Essentially, they help to activate the 'relaxation response system' and involve proactive engagement in activities aimed at inducing an enhanced state of inner calm.

Keeping an emotional diary

There are a number of studies which suggest that writing your feelings down can be emotionally beneficial. Psychologists have discovered that, for some people going through a particularly stressful period of their lives, writing a diary or journal helps to reduce their stress levels and lifts their mood.

More recently, neuroscience has provided us with a greater understanding of the brain's activity in relation to our emotions and writing things down. Research has demonstrated that, during the process of documenting feelings on paper, activity in the amygdala (a part of the brain responsible for regulating our emotional responses, especially fear, anger and pleasure) decreases significantly, and that activity in the ventolateral prefrontal cortex (the part of the brain involved in suppressing emotional responses related to negative stimuli) is significantly increased. This research suggests that, during the process of writing, the brain works to regulate the difficult emotions that are being expressed.

Keeping a diary or journal can therefore be a powerful tool in a number of ways. It can serve as a means for expressing worrying thoughts and the associated feelings. Recording those uncomfortable feelings on paper offers you a form of release by providing an emotional outlet. It helps you to avoid the pitfalls of bottling up difficult emotions which can then become too overwhelming to manage.

Setting a definite time during the day to write in your diary is best, because you then know you have a special space in which you can release the anger, frustration or fear that you might be feeling. You will know that you can do this without letting those feelings spill over into other parts of the day and get in the way of work and relationships.

Writing can also give you the opportunity to identify the triggers and negative thinking associated with your emotions, and allow you to see how you behave in response. It offers you a chance to step back and gain some perspective, and even to challenge your negative thinking. When you look back through your diary it may show you patterns and themes emerging over a period of time, enabling you ultimately to make sense of your feelings.

Mindfulness

Mindfulness-based stress reduction was originally a religious practice which evolved from the ancient Buddhist practice of meditation. It is about using sensory stimuli to focus on being fully 'in the moment' with the use of enriched awareness. At the heart of the method is a philosophy promoting being in a way that is non-judgemental and accepting.

Often internal dialogue can provoke anxiety. We tend to fast-forward into the future with worrying thoughts, delving around in uncertainty and trying to find answers that are not necessarily there.

We are also prone to rewinding the past, ruminating over situations and events we tell ourselves we could have handled better, that should have been avoidable. This type of negative thinking about both past and future can be detrimental and may contribute to our current feelings of stress. And when we continually focus our attention on past and future we run the risk of missing life in the present.

Mindfulness helps us to take control of the ruminations that contribute to stress by allowing us to focus attention elsewhere for a short period of time, to take a temporary breather from the racing negative thoughts and internal critical commentary that often seeps into our consciousness. Instead, the meditations involve heightened awareness of our bodily sensations and our physical environment, anchoring us in the here and now. It enables us to achieve an observant and non-critical attitude which helps to dispel the internal dialogue.

To practise mindfulness meditation you should find somewhere quiet and peaceful so as to avoid being distracted or disturbed by external goings-on. Assume a comfortable position (this does not have to be the 'lotus position' – just make sure you are sufficiently comfortable that you are not excessively aware of your body). Choose a point of focus, something on which to concentrate. This can be either external or internal: for example you might concentrate on a particular sound in the environment, or on something visual such as an ornament. Try to be observant and non-critical, meaning that when intrusive thoughts come into your mind just gently, and without judgement or analysis, acknowledge them and turn your attention back to your point of focus.

Yoga

Yoga is an ancient Eastern practice which aims to relax and strengthen both body and mind through the use of breathing control, meditation and placing and holding the body in different postures (known as 'asanas'). There are a number of different yoga schools, including Hatha, Ashtanga, Bikram, Anusara, Vinyasa and Kundalini, to name but a few of the most popular ones adopted in the West.

The different types of yoga all include a concentration on posture, but each also has its own particular emphasis such as pace, intensity, use of breathing, level of physical demand, or the importance placed on physical alignment and the use of chanting. The yoga postures target areas of the human anatomy such as nerves, glands and organs in order to stimulate enhanced functioning. The idea of placing the body in particular postures is based on knowledge of human anatomy and physiology. In a similar way that mindfulness entails a focus on the 'here and now', yoga requires significant concentration in order to work the body into and hold the postures. This again means that you focus on the here and now, rather than on the ruminations and worrying thoughts that may drive feelings of stress. In addition, the breathing techniques involved in yoga direct the mind to the inhaling and exhaling of breath, which can help to prevent intrusive thoughts from dominating the mind, thus providing deeper relaxation and greater release from negative emotional states.

Visualization

Imagination can be a particularly powerful tool for some people as it helps to create a mental retreat from the everyday stressors that we face. This way of reducing stress once more provides a change of focus from the flow of anxiety-provoking thoughts flooding our minds, thus offering us a little sanctuary. Visualization relies largely on your ability to concentrate and to connect with imagery designed to help you feel a greater sense of inner calm.

The most commonly used visualization techniques encourage you to use your imagination to develop a mental scene of a serene and beautiful environment, one which for you is associated with a peaceful internal state and a sense of happiness. You might, for example, imagine a place of natural beauty or a favourite room which always makes you feel safe and calm. The more intensely you are able to imagine the scene, the greater your chance of the exercise being effective, thus enabling you to achieve a greater sense of relaxation.

When practising visualization you should use your senses to make your chosen scene feel as intense and real as possible. For example, if you are imagining sitting on a remote tropical beach, you might focus your imagination on what you can see, say the turquoise of the ocean against a backdrop of cornflower-blue sky, and golden sand glittering in the sunlight. You might next focus on the sounds in the environment: waves gently lapping the shore, or the wind gently rustling through the palm trees just above the shoreline. Then you might switch your attention to what you can smell – the sea, the scent of flowers on the breeze – and go on to taste the sea salt on your lips. Gradually you immerse yourself deeply in the scene through the use of your imaginary sensory experience.

You should attempt to stay in your imaginary environment for some time, immersing yourself completely in the scene you have imagined, enabling your mind and body to unwind and relax fully. Then, slowly and gently, allow yourself to rejoin the world.

All you need for this type of meditative exercise are a quiet space and your imagination, as well as the determination and commitment to making the time for it, on a regular basis and whenever you need to retreat from your stress.

T'ai chi

The practice of t'ai chi originates from China and, although it is also a martial art and a form of self-defence, it is in essence a form of meditation that focuses on strength, alignment, flexibility, balance and breathing, incorporating both body and mind. T'ai chi has therefore become associated with both psychological and physical well-being.

T'ai chi helps to induce a state of calm and relaxation. It entails the practice of a series of flowing and controlled movements through a range of postures, coupled with breathing techniques, and requires a significant amount of concentration and awareness. Again, the focusing of the mind on the current activity detracts from the negative thought processes which create pressure and maintain stress. This ultimately gives the mind a break, helping to release the accelerator driving the uncomfortable emotions associated with stress.

Sharing emotions

For some of us, holding in difficult feelings may be a struggle in itself, and the feelings may spill over like a tidal wave, making it clear to everyone else that we are struggling. For others, it may seem easier to internalize difficult feelings and try to manage them alone, with the result that we bottle things up and become disconnected from those around us, perhaps because of shyness or reserve, or because we are afraid of appearing vulnerable – or too proud to admit to struggling with some aspects of life.

Locking away our feelings is likely to have a negative impact in the longer term. We may become emotionally numb or desensitized to experience, remote and distant from others, unable to access and express our emotions, cynical, avoidant of uncomfortable feelings, or even untrusting of other people or ourselves. The stifling of difficult emotions can also lead to self-sabotaging behaviour such as binge eating, excessive alcohol consumption, too much screen time (TV, surfing the net, video games, an obsession with internet pornography) or other behaviours that offer a temporary escape from our difficulties.

For many people, talking about what is bothering them and expressing how they are feeling in relation to any given stressful event is a powerful form of release. So it may be important to be able to reach out to others. It can allow you to release pent-up emotions, gain perspective on what has been happening and receive reassurance, and enable you to feel that you are not alone. Simply knowing that someone cares enough to listen can be comforting and helpful. Sometimes, being able to confide in a trusted friend or family member can be sufficient. Other people need, or prefer, someone impartial such as a counsellor or psychologist, who will be able to provide a contained space in which to listen without judgement and provide supporting strategies for coping better with difficult feelings. Whatever we choose, sharing our emotions with others is almost always more helpful than internalizing them and bottling them up.

When you are dealing with stress, and the uncomfortable co-existing emotions that may be involved, it should be comforting to know that there are a number of strategies you can use to deal with those emotions. The important thing to remember is that different people have different reactions, and will need and choose different methods for dealing with their stress. For some people, releasing their emotions through writing or talking to others is what is required; for others a meditative practice such as mindfulness, yoga, visualization or t'ai chi is what they need to regain a sense of inner balance and peace.

You may decide that one of the above approaches is right for you, or you may choose a combination of some or all of them. What is important is making the commitment to try out the various methods outlined in this chapter and experiment to see what works for you. Making the decision to do something about your stress rather than burying your head in the sand is certainly preferable for longer-term emotional health, so it may be a good idea to start experimenting with the methods in this chapter as your next step.

7

'Work is my biggest source of stress! Can you help?'

Countless people we see professionally tell us how, over the past five to ten years, work has become their biggest source of stress. They feel they can cope with the challenges that stem from stress at home, in their family or social relationships, or with economic stress – but at work they often feel that they have little control over the stress they experience, and this sense of a lack of control intensifies the stress. Clients or customers, relationships with colleagues and managers, professional obligations, deadlines, financial pressures, and the often ever-present fear of losing a job are all strong drivers of stress and reinforce the sense that we have no control over the source of stress or its remedy.

According to research carried out by the Health & Safety Executive, one in five people suffer from workplace stress, and the Health & Safety Commission report that cases of work-related stress have doubled over the past decade. Workplace stress, according to a survey carried out by the Mental Health Foundation, is the most commonly reported form of stress (identified by 28 per cent of those responding), even above money worries (26 per cent).

It is important to understand how stress affects you at work and how those effects extend beyond work, specifically with a view to developing methods by which you can alleviate it, reduce its impact on you and on your loved ones, and cope better with it when it does occur.

What causes stress in the workplace?

Most people who experience stress at work can identify a combination of factors they believe have caused or contributed to their stress. Some factors may be unique to an individual or to his or her particular workplace, reflecting the specific circumstances of a job, role or organization, while others may apply more generally across a range of settings and affect people at different levels of responsibility. When we experience specific stresses in a particular workplace which we find overwhelming and incompatible with our needs, values and resilience, this can trigger us to look for a job elsewhere. When, however, it is stress that can be found across many work settings we may need to question whether we are in the right kind of job or whether we are perhaps better suited to another kind of role. Or we may be challenged to find new or different ways of coping with stress so that we can improve our resilience and feel more in control of our work situation.

The sources of stress in the workplace fall into the following broad categories:

- *Working conditions*: these may relate to the physical work situation, for example an open-plan office which is noisy and disruptive or the cramped and confined conditions of a flight deck. Shift working or particular shift patterns, long hours, the need for excessive alertness, repetitive physical work, etc. can all be the source of stress in the workplace.
- *Demands of the job*: we may find these exceed our original expectations, or the personal resources to cope with the demands may be beyond us, distasteful to us, or may have palled or become wearisome over time.
- *Support in the role*: for many people their performance in the workplace is enhanced, or at least maintained, if they feel supported in their role by colleagues and managers. Support is an important source of validation; without it, we may question our value and worth to the organization, or even our self-worth.
- *Relationships with colleagues*: most jobs involve some level of interaction with colleagues and difficult feelings arise where there is a perception or experience of bullying, exclusion, or denigration by a colleague. Interaction can also be soured by colleagues and managers not having time to spend in helpful interaction because they are themselves overworked and stressed, leading their fellow workers to feel alone and unsupported in their roles.

- *Culture*: stress in the workplace may be temporary, episodic, or relate to specific staff or circumstances. However there are certain jobs or roles which are inherently stressful. A brain surgeon working in a multidisciplinary team undertaking highly specialist, sensitive and potentially life-saving work has an inherently stressful job, as has a fighter pilot operating in combat conditions. On the other hand, many jobs have stresses which are less apparent: being a yoga instructor would seem to be a job without stress, given the association of relaxation with yoga, but in fact some yoga instructors may experience stress through running their own business or constantly having to find work or students.

- *Stress at home*: while not directly related to the work setting, as we have illustrated previously in the book stress is cumulative, and therefore experiencing high levels of stress at home can make dealing with challenges in the workplace more difficult.

The effect of stress on organizations

There are several areas in which it is known that stress has a negative effect not only on individuals but on the well-being of the workforce as a whole and on the effectiveness of an organization. This is why some organizations have, in recent years, made stress management and stress reduction an important part of employee training. It is well known that stress can lead to high levels of absenteeism, which is not only detrimental to the individual but obviously also has consequences for the organization where they work. Other people will have to pick up the work of the absent employee, temporary staff may need to be employed, deadlines may be missed – any of which can lead to extra stress on other members of staff.

Stress at work can also lead to conflict between individuals working in teams, which often reduces the capacity of the team to function effectively. In addition, there are likely to be higher levels of staff turnover in organizations where stress levels are high among employees – staff may be inclined to leave for another organization with a less stressful environment. This obviously is a serious loss to any organization, given that staff are its most costly asset, but there may also be other considerations such as expensively trained and knowledgeable staff joining a competitor. Legal wrangles, which are costly, time-consuming and emotionally draining, may also create a situation where employees are under continual stress.

Physical health problems, as mentioned previously in this book, can result from prolonged stress. There is evidence that stress of this type can impair immunity, making people more susceptible to infections, and can lead to other problems ranging from skin disorders to reduced cardiac functioning. As well as affecting individual employees, from the perspective of the organization such problems can lead to higher levels of sickness.

Mental health problems – including depression, anxiety, anger and increased irritability – sometimes leading to substance misuse (overuse of medication, alcohol use and recreational drug use), or potentially harmful activities such as gambling, may result from stress in the workplace, particularly where that stress is prolonged. Such problems may give rise to enduring long-term difficulties which negatively affect sleep, confidence and other important areas of personal well-being – as well as being costly to treat.

Stress can impair task performance. It is increasingly recognized that a stressed worker is more prone to making mistakes and causing accidents – which is obviously of particular concern in workplaces where safety is critical (building sites, oil rigs and hospitals, for example). In an office setting, a sleep-deprived or stressed employee may make errors such as inadvertently emailing the wrong information to the wrong person, or calculations and forecasts may be made incorrectly and large amounts of money lost as a consequence.

Stress at work can also be detrimental to motivation. Employees under stress may feel saturated with negative feelings, drained of personal resourcefulness and creativity, and lack the desire to be at work and contribute in the way they normally would.

Finally, workplace stress can have a negative impact on personal relationships. People may find their ability to tolerate problems impaired, and their frustration threshold lowered. Feelings of anger, anxiety, resentment and low mood can stem from stress which has been generated in the workplace and over which we feel we have no control and which we are unable to handle. Sexual functioning can also be adversely affected by stress, in turn putting partner relationships under stress and, in yet another vicious circle, further increasing the stress in the relationship.

Stress and the modern economy

As we noted above, stress at work has become especially prevalent in recent years. Many people we see, and indeed many clients who visit counsellors, therapists and psychologists, report that the economic downturn of the last few years has had a profound impact on their personal lives, which in turn has been a considerable source of stress in the workplace. There are specific reasons for this, including:

- fear of loss of a job or career;
- a cap on salaries and benefits;
- lack of mobility in a job or career;
- a heavier workload where organizations have made cuts in the workforce.

Increasing automation also has a role to play as a cause of stress in the modern workforce. Fears that roles or jobs may be taken over by machines or automated processes, or be outsourced to a cheaper labour force now that the world has been electronically shrunk, are ever-present and very real.

Modern ease of communication is another two-edged sword. While most of us can enjoy the benefits of the internet, mobile phones and portable computers in our personal lives, the demands and stress which this 'always-on' communication generates in people's work lives can be considerable. Many people we see say that they find it difficult to switch off from the incessant demands of emails, social feeds, text messages and the like, which arrive at all hours of the day and night, often unexpectedly, and reach us almost instantly wherever we are. They fear switching off the devices and limiting access in case they miss something important at work which could jeopardize their job.

As mentioned, job security can no longer be taken for granted. Newspaper headlines and chatter between colleagues is an ever-present reminder to all of us of the relatively fragile standing of some jobs and roles. In spite of our best efforts to be productive and show ourselves in a good light to our employers, sometimes the worst can happen. The fear that this might be an outcome is always there for many people and is a source of stress even though – or perhaps because – it is not something which they can directly control.

In the current economic climate, some roles at work have become more stressful due to fewer resources being available for the execution of the job. These resources may be time, support from others, training, or the material or technical resources and support required to get the job done efficiently.

Specific causes of stress at work

Whether or not they are caused by developments in technology and the economy, there are many identifiable causes of stress at work. Below is a list of real sources of workplace stress about which clients have spoken to us recently. Many of these will be familiar to you. Although the list is by no means exhaustive and is not arranged in any particular order, for example by how commonly these sources of stress are reported or how pervasive the stress may be, it illustrates the wide range of stressors in the workplace, and highlights the extent to which modern work life, whether in an office, a home office, or in a job without a fixed base (such as a delivery driver or airline pilot), is subject to stress:

• Unrealistic targets imposed by other people. Such targets perhaps do not reflect market conditions or 'life in the real world', but if you make an objection on this basis you are not listened to or your objections are dismissed.
• Fearing the loss of your job or career, whether through redundancy or impending retirement; worrying about the financial implications, and also feeling profound concern about the loss of identity and status which is part of having a job and a role in the workplace.
• Worrying that work stress will spill over into another area of your life and tip things over the edge (like the 'stress bucket' in

Chapter 3), making issues in the rest of your life more difficult to deal with.

- Not having sufficient time, due to work pressure, unrealistic targets, cutbacks in staff, etc., to complete tasks properly, and therefore not gaining a sense of accomplishment and of 'a job well done'.

- The journey or commute to work, which can be difficult, tiring, unpleasant – or even dangerous, for example having to fight to board an over-full train each day.

- Clients or customers being unpleasant, demanding, rude, exhibiting a sense of entitlement, being aggressive or bullying.

- Adapting to regulatory changes, within the organization or externally imposed, perhaps stemming from the recent financial crisis or the tightening of professional regulations due to increased fears about such matters as food safety, workplace safety, personal privacy, human rights, litigation, etc.

- Conflict over scheduling between your work commitments and your personal life. For example juggling visits to a doctor or dentist, getting to a post office, waiting in for people to come and fix something or for a parcel to be delivered, with a tight work schedule. In some jobs this scheduling conflict is severe: for example, many members of the police force will talk of often missing family celebrations, and some businesspeople often find they are away from home, even in a different country, on special family occasions.

- Long working hours, giving rise to cumulative fatigue and also reducing the time available to relax and to learn and adopt ways of overcoming stress, such as yoga, meditation or a hobby. It can then feel that stress is never-ending, never properly resolved, and so escalates when you go back to work after a break. Cumulative stress raises the level of adrenaline in the body, making it difficult to relax and 'switch off', and puts the body into a form of hyperdrive to the point where relaxation becomes impossible even when there is downtime. Recreation is then no longer something to look forward to because exhaustion has crept in and there is no feeling that it will be sufficient and rewarding.

- A fear of catastrophic outcomes in the workplace due to your own handling (or potential mismanagement) of a situation. This may be due to resourcing problems and not having sufficient support to complete the task, or of course due to an actual lack of competency.
- If you are taking prescribed medication, worrying about its side-effects, which can affect mood, mental alertness and general functioning in the workplace.
- Having multiple roles or jobs and feeling that it is impossible to carry out any of them successfully.
- Working in a family business where personal and professional issues and dynamics may overlap. Even minor difficulties or a fallout with a family member can have a particularly high impact in a family business, and often a lack of privacy or the need to interact with the same people both at work and at home can add to the stress of this particular work situation.
- Worrying about taking time off work, in terms of the impact this has on your colleagues who will have to take up the slack. Or worrying about whether what happens in your absence will have a detrimental impact on your position in the organization or even on your job security.
- Being asked to do things which are unprofessional or unethical by somebody more senior or powerful at work, and not feeling you have the authority to challenge them or refuse.
- The volcanic or uncertain temper of a colleague or a boss. This and other forms of aggression can have a profound effect on the mood and confidence of anyone in the workplace who is on the wrong end of them.
- The job that you are required to do not resembling the job description to which you originally signed up.
- Inflexibility within the workplace, where old or inappropriate rules are retained and adhered to rigidly.
- Everyone wanting a piece of you, so you never feel you have enough time to complete the job in hand, or to work creatively.
- A lack of proper communication within teams. Ineffective and ambiguous communications can give rise to uncertainty and stress, and can also make it difficult to understand who is responsible for a task – which itself can increase stress.

- Paradoxically, being good at your job may lead to increased stress as others perceive you to be effective and a 'go to' person, thereby increasing your responsibilities and workload.
- Not having the authority, power or influence to effect change or even do certain things within the organization.
- Other people's personalities (for example spoilers, bullies, people who adopt a 'Screw you' attitude, those whose stress is infectious, competitive and rivalrous colleagues who are not team players but play a lone hand, people who take sides or toady to others to create power imbalances in order to fulfil some covert agenda).
- Having multiple tasks thrown at you so that it becomes impossible to prioritize.

Robert was a young commodities trader enjoying life in the fast lane and the money and lifestyle his job brought him. Out of the blue he experienced an episode on the Tube where he suddenly could not breathe, started to hyperventilate, and had to lie down on the floor of the train in his City suit, which obviously attracted a lot of attention. He felt humiliated and embarrassed and worried that people at work would find out and doubt his capabilities. He went to his GP who sent him for various tests, but these all came back negative. Robert knew he was stressed in his work because he felt he was struggling to understand exactly what he was doing – none of his family had a background in the City or even in office work: his father was a decorator and his mother a housewife.

Robert shrugged off the incident and carried on with his high-flying life, getting to the point where he was mentoring young hopefuls joining the firm. He dealt with the stress by drinking after work, using recreational drugs, and continually eating chocolate bars and sweets, and drinking cola and coffee during the day. He lived his job, staying late in the evenings, socializing after work with other traders and often going into work at weekends; the stress was continuous and he was no longer happy. The final straw came when his boss telephoned him on holiday at 3 a.m. asking him to come back to the UK and into work immediately because of a crisis which was going to affect the market radically. Robert burst into tears and finally, after several years, confessed to his partner that he could not cope any more. She immediately persuaded him to see a psychologist. After only a few sessions, Robert quit his job, downsized his lifestyle, and went into partnership with his father.

You might feel somewhat overwhelmed at this point in the chapter because you recognize only too well many of the sources of stress described. On the other hand we hope you can also gain some reassurance that your experience is similar to that of many other people in today's fast-paced world of work. And you can also be reassured that, like Robert, it is possible to find solutions to your workplace stress.

What can I do to overcome stress at work?

In today's competitive and fast-paced world, it may be advisable to take the initiative in addressing your stress in case it is assumed that you can cope with anything thrown at you. Here are some ways in which you can begin to tackle your stress issues at work:

1 Evaluate the cause of the stress: is it part of the job for which you signed up? (If you are a member of the armed forces, or a trader, then obviously stress is part of the job; if you are a back office accountant, then probably not.) If the job should not be stressful, evaluate why it is in your case.

2 Establish whether or not there is something you can do about the cause of the stress; is it under your control? (For example, is it a direct – and hopefully temporary – problem caused by the economic downturn or is it due to your team's lack of coherence?)

3 Establish to what extent your expectations, thoughts and per-ceptions of your job and your role at work are part of your stress issues. Is the dissonance between what you thought being a lawyer would be all about and the day-to-day realities of working in a law firm at the root of the problem, for example? Do you consider you should be at a senior level in your job by now and feel that you have failed or that a colleague has cheated you of the promotion which should have been yours? While it may not be welcome or straightforward to do so, you may need to consider whether the job and organization is right for you. More radical change might be the best solution.

4 Ask yourself questions about your work–life balance: do you see things out of proportion at work because work is the centre

of your life? Do you feel that everything that happens at work reflects on you personally and your standing in the world? Do you take your work home with you in every sense?

5 If you are concerned about losing your job, or about retirement, ask yourself if your fears are realistic. If you were to lose – or give up, or change – your job, what would really be the effect on you, on your family, your social standing? If you were to down-scale or downsize your job, what would be the benefits? Could you manage on a reduced income if you made changes in your lifestyle?

6 Consider whether you are getting the support you need. Do your colleagues, your boss, senior management and your family know what you do at work and what it is about your role that causes you stress? Have you explained, or have you merely complained? Have you drawn up workable, practical (even money-saving) plans and strategies and put them in front of the right people at work? Have you explained to your family in what ways you need their practical or emotional support when you are experiencing stress at work?

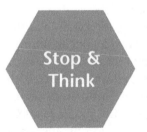

Look at the questions and suggestions above and, in a separate session for each one, write down everything you feel and think about your answers to the questions raised. Evaluate what you have written and, where you can identify appropriate action, draw up an action plan. Set goals for achieving each stage of your plan (see Chapter 10 for a goal-setting strategy).

As we have argued throughout this book, stress is not inherently bad, but an overload of stress impairs performance and physical and mental health. The worst scenario in the workplace is to feel that colleagues and employers are not taking notice of your stressed state and so fail to intervene. Outside intervention and help may be needed in this case. However, much change can be initiated by challenging the way you think about and deal with stress in the workplace.

8

Stress in family life

There is a circular relationship between family life and stress. On the one hand, simply living in a family (whatever its nature and make-up; we are talking here about 'family' in the loosest sense, not just the nuclear or traditional family) – that is to say living together with others in the same household or being part of a relationship network – has moments of stress. For many people this stress can be a powerful and ongoing feature of daily life.

Of course family relationships may themselves at times be a direct source of stress. Challenging teenagers, ageing and dependent parents and absent partners are among the many factors that may be detrimental to our happiness at home. Straitened financial circumstances, and the additional pressures these place on working parents, can bring stress into the household even when family relationships are sound and rewarding.

Equally, stress experienced by an individual, for example in the workplace, concerning financial matters, or as a concomitant to health or financial difficulties, can be brought into our families and have a ripple effect on them. Individual symptoms of stress, such as sleep difficulties, appetite changes, social withdrawal, sexual problems and many others, can spill over into family relationships, leading to secondary sources of stress. And ongoing stress can lead to marital and relationship difficulties such as loneliness, alienation and feelings of rejection – all of which may negatively impact on our well-being and the quality of our relationships.

Whatever its source, stress can put a strain on family relationships, which is ironic because we hope and expect that our family relationships will be a buffer for us against stress in the wider world. This chapter will help you to reflect on the place of your personal relationships in your life, and the connection between the quality of these and your stress.

Internal stress factors

Stress in families is similar to personal stress: there are factors both inside and outside the family's functioning which contribute to stress. Internal stressors which affect family relationships are easy to identify (some of them have already been mentioned), and include:

* not getting along with other family members;
* differences or conflict over discipline or values;
* personal space issues, which typically arise where we feel that our living space is cramped or restricted;
* conflict over friends and lifestyle choices;
* a family member consuming too much alcohol, relying on recreational drugs, gambling excessively, etc.;
* physical health problems or acute or chronic illness in the family;
* financial difficulties;
* parents or key members of the family not getting along with one another;
* bullying between family members;
* work stress which is not left in the workplace but is brought home;
* living with uncertainty (for example financial problems, long-term or undiagnosed illness, whether or not a family member is going to leave, etc.);
* absences from home due to work commitments;
* single parents being unable to rely on a co-parent to help out with major decisions, the running of the house, daily chores, etc.;
* childcare issues, especially for single parents or where both parents are working full time;
* difficulties which emanate from the extended family, such as problems with relations or in-laws;
* pregnancy and/or the arrival of a new child;
* moving home;
* separation and divorce;
* the death of a family member.

These stresses commonly occur in many families and several may be present at the same time; many can correctly be identified as 'normal' life events and situations. However, the point is that if you are experiencing just one of them it can be challenging and uncomfortable – but when more than one is present your ability to cope may well become impaired. It is easy to see how they can become overwhelming and give rise to more profound psychological difficulties.

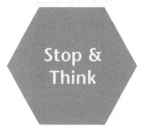

What are the main sources of stress in your family? Are they external or internal, or a mixture of both? Do the sources change, or have some of them been present for a long period? How have you addressed the sources of stress in the past, and why have such strategies not worked?

We can also identify some particular situations that often give rise to stress within the family. Let's now go on to examine these in more detail.

Stresses due to personality style

In the family, the personality of one particular member may clash with the inherent – and often unspoken – beliefs and ethos of the family as a whole. Aspects of ourselves which reflect our enduring personality and strong ideas and beliefs, and which conflict with the family ethos, can be deep sources of stress. For example:

- A belief that not relying on other people in the face of trouble shows resilience, fortitude and independence from others. Suppressing stress in this way may well itself prove stressful.
- The holding of strong views in the face of pressure, for example a parent who tells a child 'Do as I say', and has no capacity or desire to discuss or negotiate contentious situations.
- Wanting to 'live life to the full' while having little or no spare capacity to deal with unexpected events or challenges at home, meaning that anything unforeseen creates significant stress.

Some people have an enormous appetite for hobbies and other activities and/or a strong desire to look after others outside the family and home, and will ignore or override the family's internal welfare as a consequence.

* Being someone who experiences emotions at a considerable level of intensity. This can transfer to other members of a family and translate into stress. One person's intensity can spread to other family members, leading to constantly heightened stress levels within the family.

* One member of the family needing extra resources to cope with stress – such as time alone, periods of quiet, extra physical space, or even the permission to pursue stress-relieving activities – which are not available within the family home. The effect is inevitably that stress escalates and becomes either intense or chronic, or even a combination of both.

Difficulties such as these within families are not necessarily an indication of deep psychological problems. Many of them can be addressed and solved without the need for a visit to a counsellor or therapist. However, it is important to recognize that if stress does not abate normally then it may be necessary to be more purposeful and methodological about planning strategies to relieve it.

Stress and holidays

Even apparently positive family events, such as planning a wedding, going on holiday or having members of the wider family in the home for a festival such as Christmas, can be a source of stress.

One example which often arises with reference to dealing with stress in the family is that of family holidays. Expectations around holidays are typically a major source of stress. The fact that we have probably saved hard for the event and looked forward to it for a long time means that, to a certain extent, the seeds of potential disappointment have already been sown. And when families are together in what can easily become a pressured context – perhaps involving a long car journey and a shared hotel room, an unfamiliar language and food – stress can easily arise and fester. Here are some pointers and suggestions which may help you to deal with or prevent stress in this situation:

- Recognize that being together as a family is bound to produce emotional intensity. This may lead to irritability, disagreements, even fallings-out. Try to treat these as temporary events and work towards solving them as they arise. Do not hang on to negative emotions. Take being on holiday in your stride and try to recover the positive feelings associated with a holiday.
- Plan and think ahead. Avoid getting stuck in a situation where feelings of stress are a full stop in your family's relationship patterns. Think of stress as a comma: something to be understood and noted as you pass beyond it. Think beyond the present, and think of the increased well-being and resilience you will develop as a result of overcoming stress.
- Prevention is better than cure: give yourself permission to recognize that, even in the happiest and most serene families, being together in the same physical space and in an unusual situation for a period of time (and particularly away from home, where you are constrained by familiar habits and accepted customs and conduct) is bound to create some stress. Things do not need to be perfect – they simply need to be good enough.
- Try to avoid strong, polarized feelings which increase a sense of negativity and stress. A holiday is not necessarily ruined because a child has a temper tantrum, or an adolescent is moody for a couple of days, or someone is unhappy because no one wants to go along with their choice of activity.
- Keep your hopes and feelings about the holiday within proportion and build in the fact that some things will inevitably go awry. Talk openly in the family about this prior to the event – even make a family joke of it which can be resurrected during the holiday whenever something does go wrong. When something has gone wrong, harbouring resentment and strong negative feelings simply intensifies the experience, and this is likely to affect other family members negatively.
- Engage other family members in holiday-related activities, both in preparation for the holiday and during the holiday itself. Allocate tasks and duties and increase the sense of participation

and preparation. (Be careful to ensure that tasks are shared equally so that there is no sense of inequality or disproportion.)

- Try to respond flexibly rather than stressfully to challenges. If a flight is delayed, shouting at the check-in staff at the airport desk is likely only to increase family stress – and at the very start of the holiday – even though you might feel momentarily better after having relieved your frustration.

Lead the way by demonstrating how to deal resourcefully and resiliently with challenges. (Observing how other people cope with situations and adopting their techniques – or working out ways you could have handled a situation more successfully than you see them do – is one way of developing your skill in this respect and is an interesting way to spend time waiting at an airport!)

In the case of a delayed flight, for example, finding somewhere quiet for your family to sit and eat, to play a game together, or to discuss plans for when you do arrive at your destination, should scale down the stress they feel at the prospect of losing a few hours of holiday time. Just because you are not by the hotel pool does not need to mean that the holiday mood cannot begin. Think of the holiday as beginning the moment you set out from your front door rather than when you actually arrive at your destination.

Try not to buy into the expectation of, or sense of entitlement to, a perfect holiday. Things will inevitably go wrong somewhere along the line, particularly if there are long journeys and complicated travel arrangements involved. Focus on the quality of family relationships while you are on holiday together, and enjoy spending time with other family members. Holidays are not only about the destination, sightseeing, eating and drinking. They are also restorative and they provide a unique opportunity for family members to learn about each other and what makes the family tick, what are its dynamics. Holidays provide the chance to strengthen family bonds and an opportunity for the family to see itself as a unit when dealing with the outside world. Take the chance to enjoy some meaningful contact with the people you love in less familiar settings and out-of-the-ordinary situations.

Where habits from everyday, normal family life are carried over into the holiday context, if these produce stress it may well be worth talking about them in advance. For example, if a family member is prone to consuming too much alcohol and becoming withdrawn or aggressive as a result, this is not the kind of behaviour which will be conducive to a positive family holiday experience.

Where there is stress between family members, focus on the behaviours or actions which have led to this rather than putting blame on a particular individual. Personalizing causation around stress can sometimes intensify the feelings. For example, 'John, it would be terrific if you helped to wash up after the meal so that we can all get to the beach sooner', rather than 'John – you never contribute! Why don't you *ever* help with any of the chores?'

Stresses caused by separation from home and those we love

Family separations are another context in which stress can arise. They may happen because a member of the family needs to travel away from home for work or has to commute long distances, or may be a result of parental break-up. Such separations give rise to difficult and complex feelings, and the absence of a parent can be a major cause of stress for a child. Adults themselves may of course also be negatively affected by separation, and they too may need to develop methods to cope with it. Here are some ideas which can help in situations of separation:

• Ensure that there is regular communication between family members. These days, with texting, emailing, Skyping and mobile phone roaming, it is rarely the case that we are unable to communicate within the family even when its members are separated from each other. It is of course important to coordinate communication times, especially if one person is at work or there are time zone differences involved. These catch-ups should be frequent and regular, even if they are brief. Frequency of contact can help us to feel more attached, secure, and part of other family members' everyday lives. Long gaps between contact, on the other hand, can make us feel distanced and may give rise to anxiety. Frequent interaction helps to enhance the stability of our family relationships and is part of the 'glue' that bonds the family.

- You may feel pressure to be always cheerful and happy when communicating with an absent family member. This need not be the case – indeed, always being bright and 'cheery' over the telephone, Skype, etc. when you are normally a mixture of upbeat and cynical, or wittily pessimistic, will only create a sense of alienation and of things not being normal – which may well worry the absent family member. He may actually suspect that something unpleasant is being covered up, which will heighten his sense of separation and may lead to anxiety and stress. Be as normal as possible in your interaction over a distance, and if you feel unhappy or stressed or worried then share those feelings with the person who is away just as you would if he or she were at home. Sharing your normal feelings can be a source of validation and will help the absent member to feel still a part of the normal ebb and flow of family life. Of course this is also true the other way round, and the person who is away should let everyone know the bad as well as the good of her daily experiences. If everyone in the family is kept completely abreast of what is happening with each other, at the time it is happening, and is able to take part, at least to some extent, by offering advice, opinions, suggestions and so on, there will be a continuing sense of being a family even though the members are physically separated. This will also make the eventual reunion and family reintegration far easier.

- It is important to be clear and positive about why separations are necessary. Where there is uncertainty, a sense of mystique, or deception around the reason for separation, this can easily give rise to anxiety and a breach of the trust in family relationships.

- Focus on what is beneficial and necessary about a separation, rather than on the difficulties and challenges. It is also important to keep a perspective on when change will happen – for example, it is important for a child to know when he will next see an absent parent. In this way the child will be reassured that the parent has definitely not gone for ever, and will learn to trust his parents' undertakings.

- When communicating about separations, make sure you validate or talk positively about your relationship. Tell family members what it is that you love and so miss about not being with them.

And on return?

The return home of an absent family member should be a welcome occasion. However, undue pressures or expectations can spoil a homecoming. Although it is tempting to make extensive, detailed, even exuberant preparations for someone's return, these preparations must not put too much pressure on the returning family member. She may well be tired and not want lots of fuss, or to meet people outside the family, or to stay up late, or even to talk about her experiences (or hear the family's) during the separation all at once. She may have been longing for a simple, quiet, relaxed return and an early night. When you are planning for someone's return, remember that the things she has probably missed are normal family interactions – she has had different experiences while travelling away and meeting strangers, so what she is likely to want is not more different things (parties, friends and neighbours dropping in, to see new clothes or hairstyles, etc.) but the familiar (a word which, of course, has the same root as the word 'family').

Children particularly should be restrained from 'pouncing' boisterously on a returning parent or family member, and it should be explained in advance of the homecoming that Mummy or Daddy may be tired and want peace, quiet and a long hug rather than to see the new Xbox and hear all about what happened in the swimming gala. Getting children to create a picture diary while the parent is away, for example, and telling them that Dad or Mum will need time to look at it carefully before they discuss it together, can create a 'breathing space' for the returner while laying down a foundation for a good catch-up and intimate interaction a little later.

Also try to strike a balance between overburdening the returning family member with a backlog of chores – or on the other hand getting all the chores done in his absence so that when he returns he feels shut out and perhaps even redundant. During long absences, make sure that the 'hole' which the absent member leaves in the family is not gradually closed up as other members take over his or her functions. When allocating their chores to other family members, make it clear that this is a temporary arrangement, for example, and get them to hand back the chore to the absent member personally (and probably gladly!) on his or her return.

The period after a separation, when the absent member has rejoined the family, provides an excellent chance to deepen family bonds and relationships. Recounting to each other what has been happening, recalling your experiences and your reactions to those experiences, is a prime chance to gain deeper knowledge of each other. Again, letting a family member know how and why he has been missed enhances intimacy in the relationship and helps the returning member to feel an integrated and valued part of the family again.

Make sure that each person in the family has individual one-to-one time with the returning member, as soon as possible in the few days after the return. Each family member needs the chance to reconnect with the one who has been away in his or her own special way, as well as reconnecting as a family.

While it is sometimes tempting, or even easy, to view absences from the family in a negative light, there is a positive side to such separations. Bonds within the family can be strengthened as members realize how much they miss each other, and letting members know why they are missed – and hence why they are valued – is a certain way of strengthening those bonds. This helps to counter the effects of stress and builds resilience within family members.

9

What to do
if this book is not enough

So far in this book we have addressed the self-help strategies, skills and techniques you can learn and apply to help you to understand and begin to overcome your stress. By this point you will have had the opportunity to try out some or all of these and will have an idea of whether or not they are working for you.

As we said right at the beginning, there is no single 'one-size-fits-all' solution to the issue of stress: some of the methods will work for you and some will not. What works for one person will not necessarily work for another because everyone is different. The first strategy or technique you try or the first skill you learn may not be successful for you – although you may well be one of the lucky ones for whom it is. It is more likely, however, that you will need to try a range of solutions before you discover the right one. The good news is that, as everything we have described is based on tried and tested, clinically researched methods which have worked for our clients in real-life situations, at least some are likely to be effective for you.

However, at this stage you may feel that, despite trying out the various strategies, skills and techniques we have described, you are not making the progress you had hoped for in overcoming and managing your stress.

That is why we have written this chapter. It's designed to reassure you that slower-than-expected progress is normal, and does not necessarily indicate that you have a much more serious difficulty than you first thought. In case you feel that your progress is slower than you had hoped or expected, we'll look here at what you can do about it.

Some reasons why your progress may be slow

Below we explore some of the more common ways in which you might be continuing to experience difficulty with stress despite your efforts so far. The list is by no means exhaustive, but you can use it to measure your own progress and evaluate your continuing difficulties with overcoming and managing your stress. Having some understanding of why you are continuing to struggle with your stress will help you to gain a deeper understanding of how stress affects you, and how different people progress at different rates in their treatment. The chapter will end with some suggestions as to what to do if your stress persists.

Persevering but getting nowhere

You probably know the half-humorous definition of insanity (often attributed to Einstein): 'doing the same thing over and over again and expecting different results'. Be aware that you might be in danger of falling into this trap if the strategy, skill or technique you have chosen to use to address the issue of your stress is not working after you have tried it for a while. It might simply not be the solution for you.

As we have already pointed out, when you are feeling stressed – particularly if your stress is cumulative over a period of time – it can be difficult to see clearly and to make sensible or rational choices. So it is important to evaluate – perhaps with the help of a friend, family member or professional – the strategies, skills or techniques you have chosen to use to overcome your stress, to see whether or not they are working for you. Keeping a journal, as mentioned earlier, can also be a great aid in making this evaluation.

Another possible reason for not making progress with your chosen method is that, while you have taken great care to evaluate and learn it, you have not actually put it into practice. (Your stress may under some circumstances actually prevent you from realizing this.) Stress may prevent you not only from seeing clearly but also from being able to achieve your goals. You may find you have avoided entering on the actual process of dealing with or managing your stress because in itself that process is too stressful.

At some point, however, the ideas from the page, the laboratory or the clinic need to be taken into the real world and we need to test how they work for us – however daunting, stressful or even emotionally painful the process may be.

If you find that you have assimilated the ideas in this book intellectually, but not emotionally or to the point where you are actually practising them, you may need to go back a step or two so that you are not overwhelmed by your feelings. As with most psychological difficulties, it is preferable when dealing with stress to take gradual, comfortable, but determined steps forward and to gain confidence each step of the way, rather than taking giant leaps which expose you to greater stress and anxiety and potentially put you off overcoming your difficulties in the longer term. There is little point in escalating your stress and anxiety to levels that feel unbearable – you will simply set yourself up to fail and may even make your problem worse. It is better to try something else, something you may find less difficult or challenging. Then each step you take and succeed in achieving will increase your self-confidence and motivate you to take the next step.

For example, if one solution you decided to try was tackling stress at work by discussing changes in task delegation with your colleagues and outlining your intention to take your full holiday entitlement with your boss, then perhaps you have attempted too big a first step. Instead you could try scaling down your initial goal to discussing with your colleagues how they feel about the amount they have to achieve in a day, and letting them know during the conversation that you feel that your workload is stopping you being as creative in your job as you know you could be. Or if your first step was to suggest to your family that rather than taking a two-week holiday abroad this year, with all the preparation and potential for travel complications and disruption this entails, you take a series of short breaks with each family member choosing a destination, you might instead first carefully plan a surprise short break and see how the family react to this kind of holiday.

Finding that the strategy, skill or technique you chose initially does not work for you, or that you have avoided putting it into practice, does not mean you have 'failed'. You tried it but at some level you decided that it was too big a step in one go or too big a first step, or it just was not the right method for you. You will almost certainly have learnt something by this stage and all that is needed is a change of method, or a breaking down of your chosen method into smaller steps.

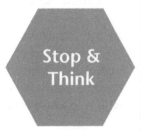

Do you think that you may have been avoiding the psychological solutions most likely to help you? Can you explain why? Perhaps you have found some of the strategies, skills or techniques too challenging? Could that be because you have attempted to tackle something too difficult to start with and need to break it down into smaller steps? Or do you need to try another strategy, skill or technique?

Procrastination

Issues of motivation can also interfere with progress in dealing with stress, and indeed in psychological therapy generally. This is not to suggest that you do not want to overcome your psychological difficulties – this is unlikely to be the case (after all, you have read this book!). Sometimes, however, it is simply not possible to give the time, focus and intensity required to overcome the difficulty at a particular point in your life. This may be because you are facing other difficulties which distract you from dealing with your stress right now. Facing up to psychological difficulties is rarely something we do in isolation – we have to continue to live our normal lives while we are tackling them.

Your motivation may also be affected by the fact that you have lived with stress for a long time. As a result you may well have developed reasonable coping strategies which allow you to avoid or manage – rather than solve – the issue. You may have become comfortable with these strategies, even though they do not provide a total or long-term solution, and this might be undermining your efforts to tackle your stress. Effectively any steps you take, or attempt to take, to change the situation and tackle the problems you have with stress take you out of your comfort zone, and so you may well find yourself procrastinating.

Motivation is also relevant in respect of the effort required of you. There is hardly any psychological issue which does not require some effort to overcome it. This is no different from gaining new skills in other areas of your life. Do you remember the first time you learnt how to use a computer? Probably you were one of the many people who struggled to find the on/off button, accidentally deleted documents or got stuck transferring files from one folder to another. In psychological therapy, the initial stages can feel awkward, stressful and almost impossible to cope with. If you are struggling to make progress, it may be helpful to reflect on and consider your original motivation to overcome your stress. You might ask yourself a series of reflective questions to assess your circumstances and motivation, such as:

- Am I comfortable in my ways?
- Is it too much effort to make the necessary change?
- Do I have the energy, stamina or motivation to overcome this difficulty?
- Are the gains I could make outweighed by the comfort I feel staying as I am?
- Could anything else in my life be holding me back from making changes in my behaviour and dealing with uncomfortable and/ or stressful feelings?

If your answers to these questions show you that there are obstacles in the way of working on the difficulties which caused you to read this book, it may be sensible to seek additional help by consulting a psychologist or therapist. Alternatively, it may be that, at least for now, the understanding you have gained by working through this book is enough.

Are you using the right solution for you?

Applying the wrong solution to the issue is a similar point to the first one that we discussed. However, it may be that although this is a *new* solution you are applying, it is still not the *correct* one, one which will help you achieve the necessary outcomes. If, for example, you keep challenging your negative automatic thoughts about a situation (as with the example in Chapter 6 of interpreting the behaviour of the neighbour who avoided you) but fail to back this up with behavioural changes (going to see the neighbour and asking if there is anything wrong and if you can help), your progress may be limited or temporary. Conversely, if you change some of your behaviour without considering corresponding changes to your thoughts, your progress may again be slow or limited. For example, if you determine to avoid catastrophizing by travelling by air although you used to avoid it because you always imagined the worst was going to happen each time you flew, getting round the problem by consuming copious amounts of alcohol before the flight to help block your catastrophic thoughts is not the answer. You need to search further for the solution which works for you.

What else is happening in your life now?

Psychological difficulties rarely exist in total isolation from other issues going on in our lives. We have partially addressed this point above; however, it is worth stressing that there may be what are termed 'cofactors' which interfere with your progress or maintain your stress. If, for example, you are experiencing low mood or you have a physical health issue such as migraine, tinnitus, a broken limb, or another medical issue which temporarily affects your ability to concentrate or function normally, then this may not be the right time to attempt to tackle your stress and make major changes in your life.

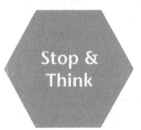
Stop & Think

What's going on in your life right now? If you are facing some of the challenges we described above, it may be that you need to tackle these before working on your stress. Make sure you're not making excuses, however, and procrastinating! A qualified psychologist, therapist or counsellor can provide additional specialist help here.

What is success?

Setting your sights on an instant and total cure for your difficulties with stress may be a bridge too far. Experience tells us that the treatment of any psychological issue can take time, even though progress is gradual and incremental. If only there were a magic pill you could take and wake up the next day completely free of all your stress! If you follow the standard psychological method using cognitive behavioural therapy, as described in this book, you can expect gradual progress towards your goal – perhaps sometimes a bit slow, but nonetheless incremental and finally successful, whether through self-help or with the aid of a professional.

Treatment, whether with a psychologist, therapist or counsellor or through self-help, requires time, patience, perseverance and a measure of determination. There may be occasional setbacks, remember, it may feel as if you are playing a game of snakes and ladders: progress seems suddenly to go into reverse, although it may quickly pick up pace again. Maintaining a positive outlook, a healthy dose of motivation, and keeping the ideas described in this book in mind will help to keep you focused and on track.

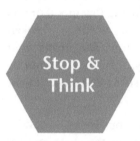

How will you know when you have successfully overcome your stress? Obviously it is never going to be the case that you will be permanently free from stress (and, as we have pointed out several times throughout this book, some stress is actually good for you), but you must establish for yourself what level of stress in your life is comfortable and acceptable in the long term. What would a realistic goal be? What level and frequency of stress will you feel happy to have in your life?

When you set goals, it is important to make sure that they are appropriate for you and a realistic possibility. When goal-setting, always bear in mind the SMART principle: set goals which are Specific, Measurable, Achievable, Realistic and Time-limited.

Getting support

If, after reading this book and trying out the strategies, skills or techniques described, you come to the conclusion that self-help is not for you, or you find it too difficult to act on the ideas suggested at this time, or if you have made some progress but now feel you are 'stuck', then perhaps finding support from a professional is the answer.

Do not fall into the trap of becoming over-critical of yourself for not having 'cured' your stress problem on your own. If you have worked through this book it is likely that you have already made progress, so start by giving yourself credit for what you have achieved. Reading even parts of the book means that you have shown the courage and motivation to take steps to overcome your issues with stress. Perhaps the act of buying the book was itself a recognition that there is an issue you need to face. At the very least, you now have more information about the nature of the stress in your life, which is a good start to overcoming it.

If your thoughts about what you need to do to tackle your stress leave you feeling emotionally vulnerable and upset, then it is perhaps time to go back to gaining a clearer understanding of these thoughts in order to explore your fundamental fear about what it is you think could happen to you. It may be that your underlying fear of some catastrophic outcome (such as being side-lined at work if it becomes known that you are over-stressed) is driving your anxiety. This may need further exploration, under-standing and targeted interventions, and can sometimes be best tackled with the help of a qualified specialist such as a psychologist, counsellor or therapist.

As we have seen elsewhere in this book, being able to share the issue of your stress with others is often an important step towards overcoming it. Friends and family members can be helpful, but some people feel unable or unwilling to share the extent of their problems with others who are close to them. If you tell your partner all about your stress, he may feel that he is in some way to blame and react with hurt or anger; if you ask a friend for help she may feel overwhelmed by the responsibility and perhaps respond by reject-ing or distancing you. Or you may simply fear this type of response, although the reality would be different. All this can make seeking help from those closest to you difficult and complex, and some people for these reasons prefer to seek help from professionals.

As we have already suggested, your starting point, if you decide to seek help from a trained specialist, could be that you have recently read this book and think, on the basis of what you have read, that you might be experiencing excessive stress. If you have been able to apply some of the ideas you have learnt in the book, you may also be able to describe why and how you feel the issue has come about and what you have done so far in order to overcome it. You could also possibly describe why you feel you are not making adequate progress in overcoming the difficulty.

We recognize that taking the issue to someone else means facing up to it and putting it in words to another person. Think of that process as part of your therapy, in that describing the difficulty and talking about it with another person is in itself therapeutic. Describing our difficulties to someone else, particularly perhaps someone who does not know us personally, is a major way of learning more about how those difficulties affect us and how we feel about them. It is an important step in bringing about change.

A session with your GP, psychologist, counsellor or therapist will help to put you back on track by assessing the nature and extent of your problem with stress and how best to deal with it and manage it. This book can then act as a companion in that face-to-face treatment. For example, you can use the book to help you think about homework exercises and in plotting your progress in overcoming your stress.

The next and final chapter has some tips and hints to help you manage your stress in your day-to-day life. It can act as a reference point and a quick reminder for you, in whatever way you finally decide to use this book – either in your self-help approach to your problems with stress or alongside professional help.

10

Tips, hints and techniques for stress management

This final chapter in the book is a practical one. Here you will find detailed explanations of the strategies, skills and techniques mentioned in previous chapters. You can use this chapter as you work through the exercises in the book and also as a checklist and reminder as you continue to work on your problems with stress in your life.

First, managing sleep. Disrupted sleep is often one of the first signs that you are feeling stressed, and can in turn exacerbate stress, so it is important that you deal with sleep issues as soon as they arise, before a negative pattern develops.

Sleep management

- *Be consistent with your sleep routine.* Try to keep a regular routine of going to bed at around the same time every night and getting up around the same time in the morning. Consistency helps your body to learn when to slow down for sleep and when to wake up in the morning. Of course it is not always easy to go to bed and get up at exactly the same times each day, but make a regular pattern the base and try not to disrupt it too often. The aim of keeping a consistent sleep pattern during periods of stress is to minimize the risk of sleep deprivation or becoming nocturnal.

- *Engage in non-stimulating activities before bedtime.* Try to wind down a couple of hours before you go to bed. Listen to relaxing music, read something light, or practise yoga, meditation, relaxation techniques, or have a massage, for example. This will help your body and mind to feel relaxed and ready for sleep. If you watch television you might find it unhelpful in terms of helping improve your sleep, as over-bright light such as that from a television (or computer) screen wakes up your body rather than relaxes it; our bodies are programmed to respond to light (wakefulness) and dark (sleep).

- *Don't eat just before bedtime.* Try not to eat for two hours (at least) before you go to bed. If your body is digesting, it is working very hard and will not be able to prepare for sleep (for example, by lowering your core body temperature).
- *Reduce environmental disruption.* Is the temperature, lighting and noise level in your bedroom helping or hindering you? If, for example, the room is too noisy try to reduce or remove the source of the noise, or consider using earplugs; if you wake up too early because the room is too light in the morning, invest in blackout blinds or curtain linings.
- *Don't use your bedroom as an entertainment centre.* If you watch television, browse the internet for long periods of time, text friends or business associates while lying in bed, this can cause your mind to associate bed with activity rather than sleep. Also, electrical humming or standby lights from electronic equipment can impinge on your brain and disrupt relaxation and sleep.
- *Dealing with worry or an active mind at night.* If you can't fall asleep within the first 15 minutes after turning the light off, try getting up and doing something non-stimulating for a short while before you go back to bed and try to sleep again. You may have to do this a couple of times before you fall asleep, and you may need to repeat the strategy for several nights before it works for you. Research has shown that you are more prone to worry or engage in problem-solving or circular thinking during the first 15 minutes of trying to sleep. It is therefore important that you try to distract your mind from worry during this period.

The breathing technique

Deep breathing relaxes the body and makes it virtually impossible for your mind to remain anxious and tense. The physical benefits of deep breathing have an immediate impact on your energy levels and your ability to deal with stress.

Here is the breathing technique, step by step. Why not record the instructions (slowly and with plenty of pauses) so that you can play them back to yourself while you are learning the technique? The technique involves taking gentle, even breaths which fill your lungs completely, and then exhaling slowly. You should start by practising in a comfortable setting when you are not too stressed or anxious. Each exercise should last for about 10 minutes and you should ideally practise twice a day if you can: once in the morning and once in the evening. Find a quiet place that is free from distractions and noise. This could be your office, at home, in the garden, or even at your local gym. When you first start practising, you may want to ensure you are alone as it is easy to lose focus when other people are around to distract you. You are also more likely to feel self-conscious if someone is watching when you practise relaxing and controlled breathing for the first time.

1   Before you start, make sure you are comfortable and relaxed. You can practise controlled breathing in a seated position with your hands relaxed on either side of your body, or lying down with your back flat on the ground. If you practise lying down you might find it more comfortable to support your back by placing a pillow or cushion underneath your knees.
2   Loosen any tight clothing and take off your shoes if possible.
3   Let your shoulder blades sink down your back, and lean slightly towards the back of the chair (or relax your back into the floor if you are lying down) to support your back. Close your eyes.
4   Start by taking a deep breath in through your nose, then exhale slowly through your mouth. Continue to breathe in through your nose and out through your mouth.
5   Try to make each inhalation and exhalation of the same duration. When you inhale, count slowly from 1 to 4, and do the same when you exhale so that you are breathing evenly in a slow and focused manner. Notice how your breathing is slowing down.
6   Feel the way your lungs gradually expand with every in breath. As you breathe out you are emptying your lungs. Your body

feels relaxed. Continue to breathe slowly, in through your nose and out through your mouth.

7 Place your right hand on your tummy and let it rest lightly on top of your navel. As you breathe in through your nose, feel the way your tummy rises. As you breathe out through your mouth, feel your hand sinking further and further down towards the middle part of your body until your tummy feels completely flat.

8 Your heartbeat is slowing down. Your arms and legs are relaxed. Continue to count slowly from 1 to 4 on each inhalation and again for each exhalation.

9 On each out breath imagine that you are pushing the tension out of your lungs. Let it flow through your mouth and out into the wider world. You are getting rid of all the tension, stress and worry.

10 Let go of your bodily tension completely. Once you feel completely relaxed, continue to breathe deeply five more times, in through your nose and out through your mouth. Feel the quiet and peacefulness around you.

11 Slowly open your eyes. Continue to breathe gently and evenly in through your nose and out through your mouth. Gently move your legs and arms. If you are sitting, raise your arms and stretch the whole of your body upwards. If you are lying down, flex your arms and legs downwards and gently move back up into a seated position.

Progressive muscular relaxation

This exercise will help you to make a distinction between tensed and relaxed muscles. Being able to do so will help you to identify when you are tense so that you can relax your muscles and relieve the tension. Muscular tension can occur automatically as a reaction to uncomfortable thoughts and to stress. We are not always conscious of physical tension, and as a result it is not uncommon for people to experience prolonged periods of muscular strain when under stress. Your increased awareness of bodily tension can therefore act as a cue for when you should use the exercise to help let go of unnecessary muscular strain.

The sequence is quite simple and takes you through all parts of your body. The exercise is best done in a lying position, but if this is difficult then sitting in a chair can work equally well. You can use the controlled breathing techniques in the previous exercise to enhance relaxation and a feeling of calm. The basic movements to use for each part of your body are as follows:

1 Tense the muscles as much as you can and concentrate on feeling the strain within your body. Hold the tension for about five seconds and then release your muscles.
2 Relax the muscles for 15 seconds and note the difference between their tense and relaxed state.

Use this basic technique on each of the following muscle groups in turn. Remember to breathe gently and evenly throughout the exercise.

- *Hands*: clench your left hand and make a tight fist for 15 seconds. Then relax your hand for 15 seconds and let it sink towards the ground. Do the same with your right hand.
- *Arms*: tense your left arm for 15 seconds. Imagine that you are holding a set of weights in your hand. Bring the bottom half of your arm upwards as this will make it easier to flex your arm. Relax for 15 seconds. Repeat the process for your right arm.
- *Face*: tense your eyebrows by frowning for 15 seconds, then tense your forehead and jaw. Relax for 15 seconds and repeat.
- *Neck and shoulders*: let your chin drop down towards your chest. Squeeze your shoulders up towards your neck as hard as you can. Hold for 15 seconds and then relax. Repeat the process once more. As your shoulders release, feel your shoulder blades slide gently down your back towards your waist.
- *Abdomen*: tighten the muscles in your stomach by pulling them in and up. Hold for 15 seconds and then relax for 15 seconds. Repeat the tensing and relax again.
- *Thighs*: relax your upper body. Tighten your thigh muscles by squeezing your buttocks and thighs together for 15 seconds. Relax for 15 seconds before you repeat the process.
- *Legs*: bend your feet downwards for 15 seconds so that your

toes are pointing towards the floor. There should be a tight-ening sensation in the back of your leg muscles. Relax for 15 seconds. Then bend your feet up so that your toes are pointing upwards. You should feel a light tension in the front of your legs. Relax.

- *The whole of your body*: tense your hands, arms, face, neck and shoulders, abdomen, thighs and legs all at once and hold for 15 seconds. You should feel the tension throughout your body. Relax for 15 seconds and then repeat the process.

Take care to not over-tense muscles as this can cause discomfort or even injury to your body. Remember to breathe slowly and regu-larly between each part of the exercise. When you have finished the sequence, relax completely for a minute or two and think about something pleasant, something relaxing which you enjoy very much. This allows a gentle transition back into your normal envir-onment. Then open your eyes and, before you stand up, gently stretch and move your arms and legs. Avoid sudden or jerky move-ments. When you are ready, take your time standing up. If you still feel tense at the end of the exercise, repeat the sequence once more.

Remember, it takes time to learn how to relax. Give yourself a chance and do not expect to succeed too soon.

Techniques for organizing your life

- One effective way of juggling multiple responsibilities is to consider your commitments. This will help to shed light on whether your daily schedule of tasks is achievable – or whether you need to rethink the way you run your life.
- Using a diary or organizer or similar (paper or digital) helps you to plan ahead so that you can organize your time more effec-tively. It also prevents you 'firefighting' – merely dealing with tasks which suddenly become urgent (often because you've left them too long!) or as they arise. Be realistic with what you want to achieve within a given time period. This will help to reduce the risk of taking on too many commitments so that you find yourself only halfway through a task by the time you are due to start the next one.

- Review, and if necessary adjust, your schedule regularly during the day, the week, the month, and so on. It also often helps to allow a day with fewer activities as this gives you a chance to catch up where there has been slippage. Allowing spare time in between tasks will also help to reduce the risk of underestimating the time it may take to complete a task.
- If you are finding it difficult to prioritize everything you have to do, try asking yourself 'What would happen if I left this till next week?', 'What if I asked x to do this?', 'Do I really want to go to that lunch/film/party?', 'Is this deadline set in stone or is there any leeway?' Looking at the consequences of postponing, delegating, outsourcing or letting go of a task may help you decide which ones are most important to you – and which ones you may be able to eliminate.
- Carry out frequent reviews of your scheduling and how well you keep to it. This will help you to see whether there is a pattern of behaviour such as underestimating time, taking on too many commitments or ignoring your scheduling when something else crops up. You should also be able to see where time is slipping away or being 'frittered'.

Goal-setting

Goals, to be effective, need to be SMART:

- Specific – if you can describe your goal in a way that defines exactly what it is, you will be more likely to know when you have achieved it and be able to see your progress towards it. 'I want to panic less' is not specific and could be demoralizing to work towards as you are unlikely to know when you have achieved it. 'I want to stop having panic attacks in team meetings' is a specific goal and you will know when you have achieved it.
- Measurable – you need to be able to measure what you are trying to achieve or, again, you will not be able to see your progress. For example you cannot measure 'I want to feel less stressed', but 'I want to reduce my feeling of stress from 9/10 to 4/10 when I commute to work/get the children off to school in the morning' is specific and measurable.

- Achievable – make sure that your goal is something that you are able to achieve. For most people, 'I want to take the whole family away to a luxury hotel somewhere abroad for a six-week holiday so we can all destress' is not achievable, whereas 'I will take the family on a short break to that little hotel in Cornwall in July and get everyone to talk about what they want to do before we go' is precise and achievable.
- Realistic – make sure that your goal is realistic given your physical abilities, practical resources and time. If your stress is related to a fear of flying, for example, it may not be possible or even useful to aim at being able to fly to Australia. However, setting a goal of flying to your friend's wedding in Scotland without getting stressed is definitely realistic.
- Time-limited – setting a goal without a realistic timeframe can reduce your chances of achieving it. Be careful not to put too much pressure on yourself, however. 'I want to stop feeling anxious tomorrow' is not a SMART goal! 'I want to reduce my anxiety on the Tube from 9/10 to 4/10 by Christmas' *is* SMART and you are much more likely to achieve it.

You might find these questions helpful in designing your own SMART goal:

- If you achieve what you are hoping for, what will be different?
- How will other people know that you have changed? What will they see you do or hear you say?
- How would you like to think about yourself?

Take the time to design your own SMART goal. You may want to ask someone you trust for help.

Assertiveness techniques

Being assertive with people around you – colleagues, bosses, friends, family, people in authority, people you meet in public – enables you to take your place in the world without causing conflict or riding roughshod over the needs and sensibilities of others. Assertiveness can enable you to put into practice the plans you have made to change your life to make it less stressful. The ability to be assertive increases your sense of self-worth and earns respect from other people, which reinforces your self-worth further. Assertiveness is a skill which can be learned. The following tips may help you become more assertive:

* Think of your own needs as an individual. Ask yourself 'What do I want/need?' when a difficult situation arises. Remember that your own needs may be different from what you feel is expected in your role as a partner, colleague, friend, etc.
* Be direct and honest when you are communicating your wants and needs to someone else. Try to use 'I' statements such as 'I respect your opinion, but I feel uncomfortable with your view on this'. It is important both to accept and respect other people's opinions and rights (and to expect them to do the same for you).
* Take responsibility for communicating your wants and needs to other people, rather than assuming that they already know or that they will figure it out.
* If you are unsure how you feel about a matter, do not be afraid to ask for 'think it through time'. Let the other person know that you are unsure about a proposition, that you will need to think about it – and let them know when you will get back to them.
* Acknowledge when you are wrong, and when you have changed your opinion, but ensure that other people know what happened and why so that they are not tempted to see this as weakness. Allow other people to do the same and acknowledge them when they apologize or explain a change of mind.
* Recognize that you are not responsible for the behaviour of other adults. (This can be difficult if you are feeling vulnerable or are interdependent with the other people involved.)
* Try to maintain positive and confident body language when being assertive. Keep an upright back posture if possible, use clear and concise statements, and maintain eye contact (without staring or locking eyes with someone in what might be seen as an aggressive way).

General tips and hints
for avoiding and preventing stress

- Take regular breaks from what you are doing. This helps to stimulate you to refocus on the task in hand, while stepping away and changing your body position and environment for a short period will refresh you physically.

- Eat as healthily as possible. How, what and when we eat has a direct effect on our mood, our energy levels, and our short-term and long-term well-being. It goes without saying that unhealthy snacking causes you to experience rapid fluctuations in blood sugar levels, which stresses the body. (For example, drinks high in liquid sugar, such as most carbonated drinks and even many commercial fruit juice drinks, may give you a burst of energy but this soon abates and you are then likely to experience unpredictable fluctuations in your energy and mood.)

- Reduce your alcohol intake (and/or recreational drug use, abuse of prescribed medication, etc.). This will improve mental well-being and alertness, allow you to feel more energized and have a more buoyant mood, and enable you to maintain a healthy weight. Alcohol is a central nervous system depressant and, while often desirable and beneficial in helping initial relaxation, ultimately it has a negative impact on sleep, mood, concentration and sexual performance.

- Take positive steps to achieve good sleep as a significant contribution to resolving your stress issues. Sleep is important for restoring and maintaining good mental health, and without deep and uninterrupted sleep stress can escalate or can seem never to abate.

- Regular exercise is an extremely important countermeasure to stress. The effect of any mildly aerobic exercise (at the very least, something like climbing a long flight of stairs or going for a power walk) helps at a chemical level to release endorphins into the bloodstream and the brain, which gives a sense of natural well-being – and even a small 'high'. Aerobic exercise also suppresses the secretion of cortisol, a hormone particularly associated with stress. This type of exercise can also help to counteract the negative effects of having a sedentary job, and in maintaining a healthy weight which, again, will help to lower stress levels.

- Having hobbies and interests outside your work – and which are very different from what you do in your job – will sustain and replenish you. We have all heard the old proverb 'All work and no play makes Jack a dull boy', and it is vitally important that we take time to 'play'. Hobbies and outside interests help to improve your contacts with social groups outside the workplace, validate other sides of yourself than those you share and use at work, and sharpen your focus by taking you out of your work zone and requiring you to learn new skills and ways of interaction. Hobbies can also be a welcome distraction from workplace problems and issues.

- Set aside time for companionship and personal relationships. This means scheduling time with friends and family and seeing this as being equally important as time spent engaged in work activities. Enjoying time with family and other significant people is beneficial to you and serves to remind you that there are other aspects to your personality than those exhibited at work.

- At work, establish boundaries to serve as proper limits to the amount of work you can reasonably be asked to cope with. Obviously such boundaries will need to be negotiated with managers, colleagues, etc., but if done positively, showing clearly that as a result we are more productive, and happier, in the workplace and as a member of a team, the need to set and observe boundaries should be respected and supported.

- Delegating to others is an important tactic in daily life and at work. A reluctance to delegate can stem from a fear that other people will encroach on your job or your standing within the community or at work, or undermine you in some way so that you feel less worthwhile or even redundant. Recognize this and let go of the need to take the world on to your shoulders and be over-controlling.

- Learn to voice your stress and distress to others. It is neither sensible nor healthy to 'carry on regardless' or to assume that other people will understand and realize what you are experiencing without telling them. Unless you communicate your stress to others, clearly and as positively as possible, you cannot expect them to understand your experience of stress and provide you with help in alleviating it.

- Take breaks and holidays, planning well ahead so that stresses are minimized, your work is covered, and people have all the information they need in your absence. (Failing to take holiday time – and even weekends – is a major cause of stress in the workplace.)
- Keep a focus on the task at hand and try not to be distracted by others which come your way in the meantime. If necessary and helpful, make a list of the various tasks you need to accomplish and assign priorities to them. Stress increases when we are overwhelmed by information or conflicting demands, leading to poor accomplishment all round and therefore to lower levels of achievement and satisfaction. It is better to do one thing completely and well rather than trying to do several things and achieving only minor levels of success with each.
- Where possible, manage your time by creating free space in your day rather than cramming every hour with tasks. Inevitably there will be overspill into the free spaces, but allow for this in your scheduling. If you start the day with a schedule which has no free space, not only will there not be time to destress, but you will also be setting yourself up for more stress by always having to run to catch up because you have no leeway when jobs overrun or something unforeseen happens.
- Try to adjust the way in which you go about managing change – this helps directly with coping with stress. If you tend to use crisis management or deal with problems spasmodically as they arise, try taking a different approach, setting specific and broader goals for stress-countering strategies. Be proactive rather than reactive to stress. Make it part of an action plan to review and adapt as you encounter new stresses. In this way you will feel more in control of stress rather than stress overwhelming you.

At the start of this book, we emphasized that stress is normal and that some stress is good and can have positive advantages. The main focus of the book, though, has been on dealing with unwelcome or overwhelming stress that can cause psychological, physical and relationship difficulties. Each individual has a different capacity for stress and we have tried to convey that we all react differently to stress, and that managing it may warrant unique and specific remedies. The starting point for overcoming stress is first to acknowledge that it is present and affecting you negatively before, second, taking practical, behavioural steps to managing it. If you struggle with either of these stages, it may be worthwhile speaking to a professionally trained therapist or counsellor who can help you to identify what impedes you getting on top of the situation, and can then support and coach you through the steps to take to help you regain control of those parts of your life that cause you stress.

Whether through self-help or professional help, we wish you the very best and all success in resolving the issue of stress in your life.

Useful addresses

If you need more assistance than can be offered by a self-help book, you might wish to work with a psychologist or counsellor. The authors of this book can be contacted via their website: <www.dccclinical.com>.

Your GP will also be able to put you in touch with reputable professionals practising in your locality.

Other sources of psychologists include the following associations: they all set standards for membership and their websites offer a search facility to find a therapist near you.

British Association for Behavioural and Cognitive
Psychotherapies (BABCP)
Imperial House
Hornby Street
Bury
Lancs BL9 5BN
Tel.: 0161 705 4304
Website: www.babcp.com

British Association for Counselling and Psychotherapy (BACP)
BACP House
15 St John's Business Park
Lutterworth
Leics LE17 4HB
Tel.: 01455 883300
Website: www.bacp.co.uk

British Psychological Society
St Andrew's House
48 Park Road East
Leicester LE1 7DR
Tel.: 0116 254 9568
Website: www.bps.org.uk

Health and Care Professions Council
(formerly Health Professions Council)
Park House
184 Kennington Park Road
London SE11 4BU
Tel.: 0845 300 6184
Website: www.hpc-uk.org

The website allows you to check whether a psychologist who has been recommended is registered with this Council in the UK.

Index